Collaborative Therapy and Neurobiology

Collaborative Therapy and Neurobiology is the book many clinicians have been waiting for: an integration of twenty years of scientific and therapeutic cutting-edge ideas into concrete clinical practices. Interpersonal neurobiology and the development of exciting new technologies that allow us to better understand the brain have provided us with an enriched perspective on human experience. Yet, many clinicians wonder how to use this knowledge, and how these discoveries can actually benefit their clients. In particular, what are the concrete practices that each field uses to help clients overcome the issues in their lives, and how can these fields build on each other's ideas? Could minimally developed concepts in each field be combined into innovative and powerful practices to foster client wellbeing? This book offers a collection of writings that provide theoretical food for thought, research evidence, and most importantly hands-on, concrete clinical ideas to enrich therapists' work with a variety of clients. Illustrated with numerous transcripts of conversations and clinical stories, the ideas in this book will stimulate the work of people interested in renewing their practice with new ideas.

Marie-Nathalie Beaudoin, PhD, a pioneer in developing practical ways of applying neurobiology, has published over thirty inspiring articles, DVDs, and books, and has been featured in AAMFT's Family Therapy. She is the founder of SKIPS and maintains a private practice of clinical and consulting services. Marie-Nathalie is an acclaimed international speaker, well known for thought-provoking and energizing presentations. www.mnbeaudoin.com

Jim Duvall, MEd, RSW, is the director of the JST Institute and has been senior editor of *Journal of Systemic Therapies* for over ten years. He is a consultant, trainer, and author who has facilitated hundreds of workshops and courses, and who has consulted with organizations throughout Canada, the United States, Australia, and Asia. He has published numerous articles, book chapters, and books, as well as co-authored a policy paper about narrative therapy and brief collaborative practices. www.jstinstitute.com

Collaborative Therapy and Neurobiology

Evolving Practices in Action

Edited by Marie-Nathalie Beaudoin
and Jim Duvall

Foreword by Gene Combs

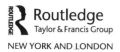

Routledge
Taylor & Francis Group

NEW YORK AND LONDON

First published 2017
by Routledge
711 Third Avenue, New York, NY 10017

and by Routledge
2 Park Square, Milton Park, Abingdon, Oxon, OX14 4RN

Routledge is an imprint of the Taylor & Francis Group, an informa business

Library of Congress Cataloging-in-Publication Data
Names: Beaudoin, Marie-Nathalie, editor. | Duvall, Jim, editor.
Title: Collaborative therapy and neurobiology : evolving practices in
  action / edited by Marie-Nathalie Beaudoin and Jim Duvall ;
  foreword by Gene Combs.
Description: New York, NY : Routledge, 2017 | Includes
  bibliographical references and index.
Identifiers: LCCN 2016045310 | ISBN 9781138655447 (hardback :
  alk. paper) | ISBN 9781138655454 (pbk. : alk. paper) | ISBN
  9781315622484 (ebook)
Subjects: | MESH: Narrative Therapy—methods | Mindfulness |
  Neurobiology—methods
Classification: LCC RC489.S74 NLM WM 420.5.N3 | DDC
  616.89/165—dc23
LC record available at https://lccn.loc.gov/2016045310

ISBN: 978-1-138-65544-7 (hbk)
ISBN: 978-1-138-65545-4 (pbk)
ISBN: 978-1-315-62248-4 (ebk)

Typeset in Sabon
by Apex CoVantage, LLC

To my husband and children who often invite me to conceive of the inconceivable.

—Marie-Nathalie Beaudoin

To my partner, Caroline, who is always standing alongside me, offering unwavering support as we travel through many journeys together.

—Jim Duvall

To all the people who love to play with new ideas, and in particular, to Michael White, who has profoundly inspired us to constantly renew our work.

—Marie-Nathalie Beaudoin and Jim Duvall

Contents

Foreword

I was surprised when Jim Duvall and Marie-Nathalie Beaudoin asked me if I would be willing to write a foreword to the book you are now holding. In recent years I have talked with both of them to seek enlightenment about what they find so interesting in "neuroscience." I have worried that all the hype surrounding pretty pictures of brains in action might be diverting time, energy, and funding away from more urgent social issues. When I told them that I still had reservations, they insisted that they wanted my reflections, saying. "We are asking you for several reasons:

- We know you and trust you
- You are a narrative therapist who is also a psychiatrist/MD
- You have a healthy skepticism of this new neuroscience/neurobiology discipline and we think that critical perspective and skepticism would add value to your forward.
- You know that we are not remotely interested in promoting the drug companies or big pharma—in fact, the opposite."

They were convincing, and I am glad they were. Jim and Marie-Nathalie have assembled an experienced and articulate team to help them share their enthusiasm for what happens when the world of collaborative therapies comes into respectful dialogue with the world of neuroscience. The papers in this collection illustrate how the emerging knowledge of mind as it forms brains and takes form in them inspires and supports new interpersonal, relational practices in psychotherapy. As I read my way through them, I developed a more nuanced understanding of how legitimating it can be for a psychotherapist to know that palpable, visible evidence of structural brain changes is taking place as a result of psychotherapy. I could also sense the excitement and innovation that come from seeing things through a new set of metaphors (amygdalas, limbic systems, mirror neurons, etc.).

In their introduction, Jim and Marie-Nathalie describe the energy and interest surrounding the conference where this book was born and give a clear overview of basic principles from both collaborative therapies and neurobiology.

Jim and Robert MacLennan, in their chapter on neurobiology and pivotal moments in therapy, use a lovely therapy story to illustrate how neuroscience information concerning memory formation can be applied to help a person get out of the "rut" of recurring negative experience and into a "groove" of hope and positivity.

Marie-Nathalie contributes a chapter on how neuroscience understandings of positive emotions can help therapists increase people's ability to move out of problematic states by cultivating counter-experiences that support counter-states. I particularly enjoyed her description of ways she helps people linger in and reflect on preferred ways of being.

Next comes a contribution from my long-time friend Maggie Carey. If Maggie finds this neurobiology stuff inspiring and informative, there must be something to it. Maggie describes the narrative therapy practice of listening for what is "absent but implicit" in people's experience. Thinking about the brain structures involved in affective processing (the limbic system) and in reflection, conscious appreciation, and planning (the neocortex) gives Maggie (and through her, us) a whole other way of appreciating and orienting to therapeutic experience.

Much of what my colleagues have found interesting in the world of neuroscience has to do with what is being learned about mindfulness practices and how they shape our nervous systems and influence their functioning. Sara Marlowe contributes a delightful chapter, sharing stories that entertainingly show how she adapts mindfulness exercises to help young children develop body awareness of their emotions, modulate "big" emotions, and cultivate positive emotional states.

Pam Dunne begins the next chapter with a riveting description of the excitement she felt at a workshop led by Dan Siegel, and how what she learned there invigorated her practice of narradrama. She gives useful examples of how dramatic enactments can strengthen synaptic connections through repetition, emotional arousal, novelty, and focusing attention.

While emotional arousal can strengthen synaptic connections, it matters what emotions are aroused and which connections get strengthened. Panic, dread, and fear can be debilitating. Marie-Nathalie has contributed a chapter addressing ways to work with the embodied aspects of strong negative emotions. She illustrates how the rich neural connections in the brain, the heart, and the gut can be altered by repeated experience, and how therapy that focuses on generating positive experiences is more effective than therapy that focuses only on cognitions.

In Chapter 7, Jan Ewing, Ron Estes, and Brandon Like contrast the metaphors of psychotherapy as healing and psychotherapy as learning. They give examples to illustrate how they focus on developing new neural networks, and how that differs from healing flawed networks. I enjoyed their discussion of "scaffolding" and how they scaffold the experience of new identity states.

Karen Young, Jim Hibel, Jaime Tartar, and Mercedes Fernandez contribute a report on physiologic research in which they measured changes in salivary cortisol and amylase, as well as EEG changes, in people who underwent single session collaborative therapy. They illustrate the importance of going slowly and carefully scaffolding new experiences in single session therapy, and share how they found physiological correlates of these changes.

The book concludes with a chapter in which Tom Strong describes his personal intellectual struggles over the pros and cons of combining collaborative and neurobiological worldviews. He reminds us that any discourse opens up certain possibilities while closing down others, and encourages us to use neurobiological discourse in ways that are flexible and that maximize resources.

I was glad that Jim and Marie-Nathalie asked Tom to contribute his chapter. It is respectful of the contributions of neuroscience while helping us to remember that all paths to knowledge are only partial paths, and that a multi-storied approach will always offer more possibilities than any single-storied approach. That said, this collection of papers sheds light on an increasingly popular and well-populated corner of the helping professions. It is chock full of inspiring examples of resourceful practice. I hope you read it with as much interest and pleasure as I did.

Gene Combs MD

Clinical Associate Professor of Psychiatry
University of Chicago
NorthShore University HealthSystem,
Co-director, Evanston Family Center
Co-author (with Jill Freedman) of *Narrative
Therapy: The Social Construction of Preferred
Realities* and *Narrative Therapy with Couples*

Contributors

Editors

Marie-Nathalie Beaudoin, PhD, is the director and founder of Skills for Kids, Parents, and Schools (SKIPS), which offers a variety of counseling services to children, parents, educators and therapists of the San Francisco Bay Area. Marie-Nathalie also maintains a private consulting practice where she enjoys working directly, or through Skype, with professionals, individuals or families wishing to untangle themselves from a variety of struggles. Marie-Nathalie has published numerous professional articles and books, including the popular *The SKiLL-ionaire in Every Child: Boosting Children's Socio-Emotional Skills Using the Latest in Brain Research*, which is written for parents, teachers and therapists, and translated into French and Spanish (*see www.skillionaire.org* for a sample of the book). She was also filmed in several Alexander Street Press videos, including *Narrative Therapy & Neurobiology: Making Changes Stick in Every Day Lives* (see www.emicrotraining.com). With a background in improvisational theater, Marie-Nathalie is an acclaimed international speaker, renowned for her entertaining and thought-provoking presentations.

Jim Duvall, MEd, RSW, is the Director of the JST Institute and a consultant, trainer, speaker and author who is recognized for his extensive practice and research involvement in brief, collaborative approaches with families, organizations and communities. He also operates an independent training and consulting practice in Galveston Island, Texas. Jim has served in the role of Senior Editor of *Journal of Systemic Therapies* since 2007. Jim is also a co-founder and previous co-director of the Windz Institute, located in Oakville, Ontario. He is the previous director of Brief Therapy Training Centres-International.

In addition to numerous articles and book chapters, Jim co-authored a policy paper entitled "No More, No Less: Brief Mental Health Services for Children and Youth" (Duvall, J., Young, K., Kays-Burden, A., 2012). As a result of the recommendations of this paper, brief core services (non-pathologizing) were mandated by the Ministry for Children and Youth of Ontario to be available to children and families in every community in the Province. His book, *Innovations in Narrative Therapy: Connecting Practice, Training and Research* (Duvall & Béres, 2011, WW Norton & Company) is the first book to integrate training and research with narrative therapy, resulting in a compelling practice evidence base.

Jim consults and trains with organizations throughout Canada, the United States, Australia and Asia.

Contributors

Maggie Carey, BA (Psych); Dip Ed; Dip Narrative Therapy, is the Co-director of Narrative Practices Adelaide (Australia). She has taught narrative therapy in many local and international contexts and enjoys the opportunity to share both the theoretical principles of the approach and the detailed practices that come from the philosophical underpinnings. Her interest in neurobiology was sparked early in her undergraduate psychology degree and she appreciates the way in which many of the recent findings of neuroscience give support to current practices in therapy. Her therapeutic work has included responding to grief and loss within Aboriginal communities; working with people who live with mental health issues, homelessness or disability; and responding to women and children who have been subjected to violence and abuse.

Pam Dunne, PhD, RDT/BCT, serves as a clinical psychologist, registered drama therapist board-certified trainer, California State University Los Angeles professor emerita and executive director of the Drama Therapy Institute of Los Angeles (DTILA) and the Creative Therapies Center (CTC). Along with authoring well over a dozen books, films, articles and book chapters, Dr. Dunne is also credited with developing narradrama, which is a specific method in drama therapy that integrates drama, narrative and the creative arts. She operates a private practice and conducts support groups and training programs, including an annual, week-long summer-abroad intensive in European locales ranging from Croatia to Scotland to Stockholm. Dr. Dunne has also pioneered drama therapy and narradrama training in both China and Russia. She is past president of the North American Drama Therapy Association and a founding member of the Board of Examiners. In 2014, she was honored with the Teaching Excellence Award in recognition of outstanding dedication to education in the field of drama therapy. A proud mother of six children and two grandchildren, she and her husband live in Los Angeles.

Ron Estes, MFT, practices, teaches and supervises marriage family therapy in community and university contexts in San Diego, California. His investigations into the inseparability of meaning-making and physical processes began while studying communication, design, art and dance in the early 1980s. A decade later, postmodern body-centered practices including contact improvisation converged with post-structuralist therapies. He learned about what has come to be known as narrative therapy inspired by Michael White, David Epston, Jeff Zimmerman and Marie-Nathalie Beaudoin. Simultaneously, his body-centered practices generated complex acts of interpretation and attention to physical states; how did *these* knowledges fit with narrative practices? Ron is a parent, co-leader of Narrative Health Initiatives, co-founder of *LIVE practice* and contributor to *Leslie Seiters/little known dance*.

Jan Ewing, PhD, became involved with narrative practices after studying with Michael White in Australia in 1994. Her clinical practice, teaching, training and research explore lifelong questions about how narratives affect our body/mind and relational practices, as well as address political social justice concerns. In 2006, she launched Narrative Initiatives San Diego (NISD), a nonprofit counseling center bringing narrative practices to low-income clients and offering trainings to persons interested in narrative. She also founded Narrative Health Initiatives (NHI) in collaboration with an integrative medical center. Here, she collaborates with a growing *practice community* of therapists and medical providers to advance an understanding of how narrative *relational practices* shape identity states and health. She has directed three university clinics focusing on narrative therapy, including San Diego State University, where she is a full-time faculty member in the MFT program.

Mercedes Fernandez, PhD, is an associate professor of psychology and director of the graduate program in experimental psychology at Nova Southeastern University (Fort Lauderdale, Florida). As a clinical neuropsychologist, she studies brain-behavior relationships. Her current research focus is in the area of experience-dependent neuroplasticity in humans.

Jim Hibel, PhD, is a family therapy professor at Nova Southeastern University (Fort Lauderdale, Florida). He serves as a special sections editor for JST. Jim practices, teaches and supervises narrative work, and has published and presented internationally on narrative teaching and training. He is the PI on a research project investigating the relationship between narrative conversations and physiological markers, including EEG patterns.

Brandon Like has been a member of the narrative health initiatives community since 2014. He regularly implements biofeedback and neurofeedback into his counseling work. He holds an MS in counseling from San

Diego State University, and is currently employed in both psychiatric and integrative health settings. He is interested in how neuroscientific research is changing both the field of psychotherapy and national public health policy. He lives in San Diego, CA with his wife, Dana, and spends as much time outdoors as possible.

Robert Maclennan, MA, RP, is a psychotherapist in private practice in Toronto, Canada. He trained in relational psychotherapy with the Creative Healers Institute, where he later served as an assistant instructor, and studied collaborative psychotherapy at the Hincks-Dellcrest Centre, where he developed a passion for neuroscience. His graduate degree at the University of Western Ontario focused on medieval religious literature and informed his earlier career as an editor and publisher.

Sara Marlowe, MSW, RSW, is a clinical social worker, children's author, university lecturer, musician and mindfulness practitioner and teacher. She has developed and facilitated numerous mindfulness programs for children, adolescents, parents and families in mental health, educational and community settings. Sara has a private counseling practice where she works collaboratively and creatively to support children and families to move towards their hopes, dreams and preferences for their lives. She is the author of two children's books. The first, *No Ordinary Apple: A Story about Eating Mindfully*, playfully teaches mindful awareness to children through the process of eating an apple. Her latest book, *My New Best Friend*, teaches children how to be compassionate towards themselves. Sara lives in Toronto with her partner, their two children and a ginger cat named Chutney. She can be found online at www.mindfulfamilies.ca.

Tom Strong, PhD, is a professor and counselor-educator at the University of Calgary who researches and writes on the collaborative, critically informed and practical potentials of discursive approaches to psychotherapy. Author or co-author of over 100 articles and chapters, he is co-author (with Andy Lock) of *Discursive Perspectives on Therapeutic Practice* (Oxford University Press) and *Social Constructionism: Sources and Stirrings in Theory and Practice* (Cambridge University Press), as well as *Furthering Talk* (with David Paré; Kluwer/Academic). For more details on Tom and his research, please consult http://www.ucalgary.ca/strongt.

Jaime Tartar, PhD, is an associate professor of behavioral neuroscience and psychology at Nova Southeastern University (Fort Lauderdale, Florida). She is widely published in many areas of psychology and neuroscience with topics ranging from clinical neurological impairments to basic cell physiology.

Karen Young, MSW, RSW, is the director of the Windz Institute, operated by the Centre of Learning with Reach Out Centre for Kids (ROCK). She is an institute faculty teaching many of the Windz workshops and certificate programs. She provides supervision to interns, organizes and designs training, oversees research projects and, for over 14 years, has supervised and provided single session therapy at the ROCK walk-in therapy clinic. Karen has provided consultation and clinical training to many organizations in Ontario, across Canada, and internationally regarding re-structuring service pathways to include brief services such as walk-in clinics. She has been teaching narrative and brief narrative therapy for over 25 years and is a therapist with 30 years of experience working with children and families. Karen has contributed numerous publications regarding applications of brief narrative therapy and research in brief services and walk-in therapy. She co-authored the *Brief Services Online Course* for CMHA Ontario (Duvall, J. & Young, K., 2015) and the Brief Services policy paper for the Ontario Centre of Excellence for Child and Youth Mental Health (Duvall, J., Young, K., Kays-Burden, A., 2012), entitled *No More, No Less: Brief Mental Health Services for Children and Youth*. Karen was the lead in the first in Ontario *Brief Services Evaluation Project, 2014*, a multi-organization evaluation of brief services.

Acknowledgments

Collaborative Therapies and Neurobiology arises out of years of rich discussions, intriguing questions and inspiring ideas with many people.

This book would not have been possible without its wonderful contributors. We have enjoyed the stimulating back-and-forth process of reading, questioning, reviewing and at times talking on the phone involved in crafting the chapters. We have all learned a great deal from each other!

We have both been involved in teaching for a long time, and workshop participants have a way of raising the most interesting questions that stretch our minds. We are grateful for those, and hope that this book will continue stimulating possibilities and imagination.

Our editor Elizabeth Grabber provided an incredibly supportive environment that nurtured a burgeoning project into an actual book. We are very thankful for her open-minded and flexible approach.

Last but not least, we appreciate the encouragements and day-to-day support provided by our respective life partners! Marie-Nathalie would like to thank her husband Paul for his loving presence on all fronts of life, and Esther for keeping everyone fed and organized during the school year! Jim would like to thank his partner Caroline for her constant encouragement and unwavering support.

Introduction
Merging Soft and Hard Sciences

Marie-Nathalie Beaudoin and Jim Duvall

Collaborative Therapy

As a therapist, trainer and journal editor I (JD) had been steadfastly committed to practicing various forms of collaborative therapies for many years. Then, a few years ago, I noticed a new and unusual movement in the field, which was the interest in linking collaborative therapy with new discoveries in brain science. Students in our training courses began submitting papers addressing the linking of collaborative therapy and neuroscience. Some were claiming that the new discoveries in brain science were, in fact, validating the practices of collaborative therapies. Our journal began receiving submissions addressing the integration of collaborative therapies and neuroscience. More and more the linking of these ideas became a controversial topic in conversations among colleagues throughout the United States and Canada. Many of us questioned this new and unusual initiative. How could this be? The notion of linking collaborative therapy, which is embedded in a backdrop of postmodern and social constructionist theory, with what we understood to be a modernist, hard science approach seemed like mixing ice cream and mustard together. Both interesting and compelling on their own; however, when combined, the result can be a strange dish. Yet, many of my respected colleagues remained compelled by the recent neuroscience discoveries and the promise for moving our work in collaborative therapies into new territories. Many noticed conceptual similarities and links, suggesting the possibility that the new discoveries in neuroscience could contribute to our work in collaborative therapies.

These conversations grew to a groundswell of stories from innovative practices that combined the two worlds. Research projects were springing up utilizing equipment that would monitor the brain activity of both the therapist and client(s) pre-, during and post-therapy session. The collaborative therapy conversations and specific questions seemed to be influencing brain activity, not only with the clients, but with the therapists as well. Thus, the importance of the relational aspect of the therapeutic conversation was underscored.

Of course, there were and remain the voices of skepticism, quick to warn us not to create a theory of the brain, and once again succumb to the "medical model" to control the art of the therapeutic process. This skepticism is, in fact, the underpinnings of solid critical theory, calling into question these new knowledges and practices as they are emerging, offering clarity and rigor as it takes shape and form.

Finally, in 2012 the conversations and experiences from practice and research had continued to grow substantively. After consulting with colleagues, it appeared to be an important time to create a forum to bring together the various practitioners and researchers with the purpose of sharing their current work and facilitate discussion regarding the emergent developments in innovative practices and research projects that were addressing and linking collaborative therapies and neuroscience.

In April 2014, we produced a conference in Toronto, Ontario entitled "Innovative Therapeutic Practices and Interpersonal Neurobiology." Dan Siegel presented the first day of the conference on his latest work in interpersonal neurobiology and the notion of the social brain. The second and third day was a conference format of inspiring keynote presentations and concurrent workshops. Theoreticians, practitioners and researchers from throughout the United States and Canada came together to share their ideas, projects and innovative practices. Some projects were completed and well polished. Some were half-baked and still in the oven, in an exciting stage of development. There were over 450 participants in attendance. The excitement was in the air. In addition to the many exciting presentations, the hallway discussions were charged with energy and curiosity.

This conference and the events leading up to it provided the inspiration to produce this book about the groundbreaking integration of hard science with the art of therapy and the implications for emerging practices.

But first, let's understand what we mean when we use the term "collaborative therapy."

What is Collaborative Therapy?

Rather than a particular model of therapy, collaborative therapy as we refer to it describes a range of therapeutic approaches that share a robust client-centered philosophy about people and how they change (e.g., solution-focused brief therapy, narrative therapy, collaborative dialogical therapy, etc.), These therapeutic approaches are non-normative and non-pathologizing, as well as situated within a postmodern and social constructionist backdrop. A collaborative therapy approach "avoids slipping into well-established traditions of thinking and talking about persons as 'disordered'." The therapeutic conversations "break free of habitual patterns of deficit-focused talk, honing in on versions of identity that foreground person's values and intentions" (Pare, 2011).

Rather than a normative standard defining what is a "healthy" identity, a collaborative approach acknowledges that there are multiple realities, people's lives are multi-storied and there exist numerous possibilities for performing identity. The philosophy, values and ethics of this approach are socially constructed and "have been historically, culturally, contextually, communally and linguistically created" (Anderson, 1990).

Therapeutic Posture and Relationship

It is worth noting that the word "collaboration" risks being a term that can be understood as contemporary rhetoric, representing a broad definition of the term that many aspire to in their practice. The collaboration we are referring to is not confined to that definition. We are proposing to take collaboration out of rhetoric and to "do" collaboration. We are suggesting that collaboration be put to work as an on-the-ground relational practice with the people who consult us.

The strong philosophical underpinnings inherent in collaborative practices provide a platform for working *with* people in partnership toward the development of their hopes for a better future. The de-centered but influential posture of the therapist is a key factor that contributes to a therapeutic relationship working productively with people to produce preferred therapeutic outcomes. Through this relationship, the therapist actively uses listening skills in particular ways, such as listening in ways that separate the person from the problem, reducing the amount of shame and frustration experienced by them. This may help the therapist to get to know the person away from the problem and, in doing so, discover what skills and abilities they may bring to bear to address the problem.

An important aspect of the therapist's posture is curiosity. It's a particular kind of curiosity that is in search of meaning. It's about being curious about people's values and conscious purposes. Through this curiosity, a collaborative therapist brings a particular orientation to a therapeutic conversation. They focus on people's abilities rather than their deficits, their strengths rather than their weaknesses, their possibilities rather than their limitations. This represents a paradigm shift away from an over-focus on what is *wrong* in people to an attentive focus on what is *strong* in people.

The "posture" or way of being in the therapeutic relationship could likely include the following:

• Being respectful and welcoming, a "host";
• Transparency and openness (including writing practices);
• Non-expert, not-knowing position;
• Collaborative, a partnership, co-authored conversations;
• Influential, but not central;
• Taking responsibility for facilitating the conversation;

- Engaged in thinking outside of what is routinely thought;
- Situated away from taken-for-granted ways of thinking;
- Interested in the details of people's experience; and
- Curious about meaning, values, commitments, hopes, dreams.

Language-Based Approach

Collaborative therapy is a language-based approach. In my (JD) research with Laura Béres we stated: "Our field research inspired us to reflect much more critically about the use of language within therapeutic conversations" (Duvall & Béres, 2011). The works of contributors such as Anderson (1997), Delueze (1994), Delueze and Parnet (2002), Derrida (1974, 1978, 1991), Foulcault (1965, 1980, 1997), and Goolishian and Anderson (1987) have contributed greatly to our understanding of the complexity and fluidity of the social construction of meaning through the words we use (Duvall & Béres, 2011). This understanding makes evident the significance of privileging the voice of the "teller" of the story. This becomes an ethical concern as we become more aware of how we use language in our conversations with people and how we talk with others about them. Michael White (1995, 2007) emphasized the need to be careful and precise in our use of language with the people who consult us. We need to ensure that we intentionally use the words and phrases of those people rather than interpreting what they say. In doing so we want to be particular about which words to pay attention to as we support the development of preferred storylines. For example, an over-focus toward gaining certainty through words and phrases that appear to represent "facts" may lead to a more linear, problem-focused and, thus, problem-solving (fixing) conversation. In contrast, a tolerance for ambiguity and tentativeness, while choosing words and phrases that are metaphorical and evoke imagery, may invite people into more reflective positions and lead to more possibilities for preferred movement.

Conversation

Because this is a language based approach, it is reasonable to assume that conversation is the central medium for conducting collaborative therapy. Based on the notion that what people bring to the therapeutic process (e.g., their language, culture, abilities, local knowledges, commitments, hopes and dreams—that is, their story) count more than any other factor toward desirable outcomes (Lambert, 1992; Lambert & Bergin, 1994; Miller, Duncan, & Hubble, 1997) in the therapeutic process, then the therapeutic conversation becomes the medium for eliciting and bringing forth people's stories. A typical linear, question-answer interviewing method closes down space for the person seeking the consultation to fully express their story. Conversation creates dialogical space for people to come forward and fully express their life events and experiences in an effort to make sense of their current situation. The quality and quantity of their participation and involvement are also strong predictors of desirable therapeutic effects. The conversational process between the therapist and people seeking consultation makes it possible to co-create new knowledge. This may be in contrast with normative, unified notions of professional, expert knowledge, which remains located outside of the therapy room and is situated within the realms of theory. Practitioners often experienced a gap between the rules of the theories they were taught and the lived experience of the practices in which they worked (Fook, 1999; Fook & Gardner, 2007; Schon, 1983).

A collaborative conversation leaves dialogical space for people to step into the conversation, while they reconsider, imagine, and realize different options and possibilities for action.

Collaborative theory is summarized in the following way:

- What people bring to the process, their story, counts significantly toward positive therapeutic outcomes.
- Therapists and people seeking consultation form a therapeutic relationship and conversational partnership.
- Relational expertise—people are the experts about their own lives. Therapists bring their facilitation skills to the process.
- Position of curiosity and fascination about various aspects of people's lives.
- Transparency—the therapist is open with their thoughts.
- Ambiguity and tentativeness—the therapist privileges ambiguity and remains careful and tentative with questions.

Why Such Excitement about the Brain, Neuroscience and Neurobiology?

In the last two decades, the subject of the brain has escaped from the confine of medical schools to books on the bedside table of many avid readers. Why are so many people suddenly interested in better grasping the functioning of this three pounds of tissue we carry around with us every day? Well, for the same reasons we seek to comprehend the meaning of life and how our food is digested, but also because the revolutionary invention of the fMRI in the mid-1990s has opened the door to greater understandings! The fMRI allows scientists to view the complex processing of the brain in *action!* This spectacular improvement in technology has allowed scientists to get a better sense of what happens when people do a mental task or process an emotional experience. For example, what happens in the brain of research participants told to subtract 17, twenty times in a row, from 20,679, and informed that this will reflect their IQ? As people go from determination to frustration and discouragement about the task (before the lack of connection with their IQ is revealed), various areas of the brain undergo an increase in blood flow and oxygenation which allows experimenters to visually witness the internal unfolding of human experience. While readers may wonder about the usefulness of some of these studies, many findings actually provide us with an insider's view of how change is possible. For example, could we learn to better understand at which point someone's description of a sad event transitions from a useful processing to one which is re-traumatizing and overwhelming?

With neuroscientists unwrapping an abundance of scientific gifts on a weekly basis, as if going through a never-ending Christmas celebration, many scientific fields have emerged and taken their place in the spotlight. Of all the branches of neuroscience now available, interpersonal neurobiology has become of greatest interest for mental health professionals.

Interpersonal Neurobiology

The growing field of interpersonal neurobiology (IPN), pioneered by Daniel Siegel in the 1990s, has been celebrated by mental health professionals for many reasons. First, while the field was still in infancy, Siegel recruited scientists from a number of disciplines in a collaborative effort to define the mind, a concept everyone used without agreeing on its meaning. After much debate, he proposed a working definition which is now well accepted in multiple disciplines from anthropologist to linguists, psychologists and physicists: "the mind is an embodied and relational process that regulates the flow of energy and information" (Siegel, 1999).

Second, after defining the mind in a revolutionary and broad way which combined physiological and relational dimensions, Siegel continued to further unite the "objective" world of neuroscience and subjective aspects of human experience. The timing of his theory was perfect. As he was writing on the interconnectedness between the brain and the environment, neuroplasticity (the brain's malleability), which had been suspected by many scientists and philosophers throughout history, became officially acknowledged in the scientific community (Lazar et al., 2005). Relationships and lived experiences were finally recognized as being both shaped by, *and shaping of*, the brain. While improved technology provided the scientific proof, interpersonal neurobiology offered a seductive theoretical framework organizing this body of knowledge (Siegel, 2007). People have intuitively known for a long time that relationship and experience matter, but it has been exciting to realize that these important aspects of human life also physiologically shape the brain in measurable ways!

Third, Siegel and other medical doctors joining the ranks of IPN defined health as involving "differentiation" and "linkage" (Cozolino, 2002; Schore, 2003; Siegel, 2007). Differentiation refers to mental structures being able to specialize in certain functions, while linkage refers to the connection of these processes with each other (Siegel, 2007). While it is beyond the scope of this section to go in depth about this concept, we will mention that Siegel has identified eight domains of integration, of which the most known are vertical-horizontal and left to right; for example, when the left brain is able to put words to right brain experiences, when important bottom-up sensations from the body are felt and acknowledged in realistic ways, and when top-down mental interpretations and memories can differentiate past-present, self-others perspectives. In other words, integration is about opposing and distinct processes becoming specialized and linked. This concept is used on a physiological level but also applied to wellbeing in families, whereas young people are understood as "needing" to separate as individuals while also maintaining a connection with their parents.

Fourth, since the mind was defined as embodied, and relationships were recognized as significant in shaping the brain, Siegel (2009, 2010) expanded his IPN theory with another key concept: "the triangle of wellbeing." Simply put, the mind influences the brain, which affects relationships, which in turn affect the mind. The triangular interaction between these three concepts reflects how the mind can regulate both the brain and relationships. This is a connection with collaborative therapies since the mind (the medium of therapeutic conversations) can modify and monitor states of being, behaviors, cognitions, and affect, and is understood as emerging from the interactions in the system (Siegel, 2009, 2010).

Finally, through his work with a family where the mother endured brain damage in a car accident, Siegel became fascinated by the overlap between functions of the prefrontal cortex and secure attachment. He eventually identified nine functions of the prefrontal cortex which have become important aspects of his therapeutic interventions:

- body regulation (balancing different branches of the autonomic nervous system);
- attuned communication (mindful presence in communicating with others);
- emotional balance (ability to be aroused but not flooded);
- response flexibility (thinking before responding rather than reacting);
- fear modulation (ability to calm oneself);
- empathy (understanding of others' emotional experience);
- insight (ability to be aware of one's own experience);
- moral awareness (attention to the larger good of the community); and
- intuition (awareness of input from embodied senses, gut and heart brain).

These key concepts in IPN have sparked the curiosity of many therapists looking to energize their practices with fresh ideas. Can IPN and CT be effectively combined?

Combining Neurobiology and Collaborative Therapies

Surprisingly, very few books and articles offer specific clinical practices, and conversational maps, which clinicians can import into their work settings. As discussed earlier, collaborative therapies, growing in popularity since their development in the 1990s, offer a wide array of specific therapeutic practices which are supported and can be enriched by recent scientific findings. Interpersonal neurobiology (IPN) offers extensive knowledge of the brain but only a handful of clinical practices to foster wellbeing. Both fields would benefit greatly from expansion using each other's ideas.

Collaborative therapies and interpersonal neurobiology facilitate therapeutic journeys in both similar and different ways. They are similar in valuing relational aspects of therapeutic conversations, using some form of externalizing language, defining wellbeing and conceptualizing identity. They are different in conversational focus and structure, therapist positioning, epistemological understandings of human experience and clinical practices.

Main Similarities

1. Therapeutic Relationship

Interpersonal neurobiology (IPN) and collaborative therapies (CT) consider relationships as a key element of the therapeutic journey. Practitioners of IPN believe that therapists' kind, attentive listening will in and of itself "heal" implicit painful memories. The re-telling of painful events which negatively overwhelmed an individual is assumed to benefit from being heard and regulated by the therapist's calm and compassionate demeanor. Because of the mirror neuron system, which allows a person to feel what another is experiencing, the complementarity of the client's limbic system's intense negative affect coupled with the therapist's right brain compassionate regulation is believed to facilitate the integration of the experience.

Practitioners of CT are also committed to a compassionate and caring listening of their clients' accounts of struggles, and have developed artful distinctions between when and how listening to a story is beneficial. For example, and as discussed earlier, much has been written on therapists' positioning and how to be de-centered and influential in listening to clients' accounts. The relationship is viewed as a collaborative endeavor in which therapists express their support and compassion by carefully paying attention to language and what is *strong/preferred* in people, as well as selecting questions fostering new perspectives and experiences of agency.

2. Externalizing Language

Interestingly, both IPN and CT use language that externalizes aspects of problems outside of people's identities. While this is practiced with a different theoretical underpinning and intention, it has the common effect of freeing clients from self-deprecation and empowering families to become a team. IPN will externalize brain structures and discuss with clients how their amygdala or their child's limbic system is getting them to overreact in problematic ways. Conversely, CT will explore with their clients how their "mad feelings" are getting them to engage in behaviors that are incongruent with their preferred selves and values (White & Epston, 1990). IPN externalizes the brain all together; CT externalizes the experience of the brain. In both cases, clients are encouraged to become an observer to their experience; understand the who, what, where, when, why of these reactions; and develop alternative ways to respond that are more congruent with their preferences. While this similarity is obvious when looking at clinical transcripts from each field, collaborative therapists' use of externalizing language reflects a philosophical stance and therefore extends beyond their understanding of problems and into the more complex social construction of identity. CT externalization is often experienced as empowering. IPN "externalized language" requires caution so that clients do not feel disempowered and governed by a brain structure, as discussed in the last chapter of this book.

3. Wellbeing

As discussed above, interpersonal neurobiologists view wellbeing as a state of integration between left and right brains, as well as bottom-up and top-down processes. In order to help clients reach a state of wellbeing, IPN will often combine compassionate listening to the teaching of mindfulness meditation. Mindfulness meditation has been found to not only increase people's awareness of the chattering in their minds and the sensations in their bodies, but it also strengthens the connective fibers in the brain which allow the frontal lobe to better regulate the firing of the limbic system. In other words, mindfulness meditation enhances awareness, regulation and access to more peaceful, satisfied states of mind.

Collaborative therapists conceptualize wellbeing as an experience of living in ways congruent with personal values supported by meaningful and reciprocal connections to others (past or present), and of being witnessed in one's preferred way of being. The process of reaching a state of wellbeing often involves deconstructing socio-cultural and political discourses, which shape how people experience themselves and others.

Both fields, in their unique ways, view wellbeing as resulting from sorting, differentiating and linking experiences. IPN focuses on vertical and horizontal information processing in the physiological matter of the brain, while CT focuses on the vertical (past and future) and horizontal (contextual and discursive) experiences of human connections.

4. Identity

Practitioners of IPN and CT define the concept of identity in similar ways. IPN would state that "[w]e are not a single self but instead a collection of states of mind" (Badenoch, 2011) while CT, in the postmodern tradition, might say that "[p]eople have multiple identities reflecting the many relationships which have shaped their lives" (Gergen, 2011). The first acknowledges a neurological phenomenon while the second recognizes a socio-cultural influence. In clinical practice, these premises allow clinicians to treat problem experiences as being only one of many possible ways of being and to not totalize their clients' identity(ies) as static and permanent.

Main Differences

While these similarities allow the fields of collaborative therapies and IPN to explore the crisscrossing of ideas and expand their respective practices, there are of course a number of theoretical differences. Since these interesting differences invite questions and debates, which will be discussed more thoroughly in our last chapter, we will only summarize three main differences here.

1. Conversational Focus and Structure

While IPN focuses on understanding the details of a traumatic event and teaches specific coping skills, CT tends to highlight people's micro and macro gestures which reflect agency, emphasize their implications and ascribe meaning to efforts. More specifically, in CT, all listening is not considered equal. Collaborative therapists often practice what Michael White (2007) has coined "Double Listening"—that is, listening for problem-related descriptions but also skills, efforts, values and preferences. Whereas interpersonal neurobiologists will prompt for details of problematic events to allow implicit memories to be articulated and understood (Badenoch, 2011), collaborative therapists will carefully craft questions which will eventually deconstruct existing problem-related meaning and their contextual component (including cultural and relational), and open space for preferred experiences of oneself. The work often involves simultaneously weaving broader perspectives of the problem and extracting specific moments of efforts, skills, agency and preferences which reflect important personal values. Since no one tolerates suffering passively (White, 2007), clients are encouraged to describe their big and small resistance to problematic experiences in a way which leaves them feeling capable agents in their lives.

2. Therapist Positioning

As discussed earlier, collaborative therapists value working with people in partnership towards living a more satisfying life. This de-centered and influential position requires curiosity and a profound belief in people's abilities to overcome their struggles. As a result, collaborative therapists will rarely teach skills, as is consistently done in IPN, but rather bring attention to efforts and highlight burgeoning moments of feeling and acting in preferred ways. Paying attention to preferred experiences, using artful clinical maps, has been found to bring forth significant changes in people's lives.

3. Clinical Practices

At this time, the main clinical practices used in IPN involve listening, providing a "corrective emotional experience" and educating clients about brain structures or mindfulness meditation. An extensive amount of clinical practices and maps have been developed in collaborative therapies. The large number of specific practices to bring forth clients' experiences of agency can ultimately be one of the major contributions of CT to IPN. One field contributes empirical finding, the other contributes clinical maps, the combination of the two yields new and fresh possibilities for everyone!

How then can we combine CT and IPN in a way that would allow mental health professionals in a variety of work settings to enhance the effectiveness and possibilities inherent to therapeutic conversations? Inspiring ideas arising from this promising marriage will be detailed in each chapter of this book!

References

Anderson, H. (1997). *Conversation, language and possibility: A postmodern approach to therapy.* New York, NY. Basic Books.

Anderson, H., & Goolishian, H. (1990). Beyond cybernetics: Comments on Atkinson and Heath's "Further thoughts on second-order family therapy." *Family Process, 29,* 157–163.

Badenoch, B. (2011). *The brain-savvy therapist's workbook: A companion to being a brain-wise therapist.* New York, NY: W. W. Norton & Company Inc.

Cozolino, L. (2002). *The neuroscience of psychotherapy.* New York, NY: W. W. Norton & Company Inc.

Deleuze, G. (1994). *Difference and repetition.* New York, NY: Columbia University Press.

Delueze, G., & Parnet, C. (2002). *Dialogues II.* New York, NY: Columbia University Press.

Derrida, J. (1974). *Of grammatology.* Baltimore, MA: John Hopkins University Press.

Derrida, J. (1978). *Writing and difference.* Chicago, IL: The University of Chicago Press.

Derrida, J. (1991). *A Derrida reader: Between the blinds.* New York, NY: Columbia University Press.

Duvall, J., Béres L. (2011). *Innovations in narrative therapy: Connecting practice, training and research.* New York, NY: WW. Norton & Company.

Fook, J. (1999). *Transforming social work practice: Postmodern critical perspective*. East Sussex, UK: Psychology Press/Routledge.

Fook, J., & Gardner, F. (2007). *Practising critical reflection: A resource handbook*. Berkshire, UK: Open University Press/McGraw Hill.

Foucault, M. (1965). *Madness and civilization*. New York, NY: Pantheon Books.

Foucault, M. (1973). *The birth of the clinic*. New York, NY: Routledge.

Foucault, M. (1980). *Power/knowledge*. New York, NY: Pantheon Books.

Foucault, M. (1997) *Ethics: Subjectivity and truth*. New York, NY: New Press.

Gergen, K. (2011). *Relational being: Beyond self and community*. London: Oxford University Press.

Goolishian, H., & Anderson, H. (1987). Language systems and therapy: An evolving idea. *Psychotherapy: Theory, research, practice, training*, 24(3S), 529–538. New York, NY: American Psychological Association.

Lambert, M. (1992). Psychotherapy outcome research. In J. C. Norcross & M. R. Goldfried (Eds.), *Handbook of psychotherapy integration* (pp. 94–129). New York, NY: Basic Books.

Lambert, M., & Bergin, A. (1994). Therapist characteristics and their contribution to psychotherapy outcome. In A. E. Bergin & S. L. Garfield (eds.). *Handbook of psychotherapy change* (4th ed.). New York, NY: John Wiley & Sons, Inc. (Original works published 1983).

Lazar, S. W., Kerr, C. E., Wasserman, R. H., Gray, J. R., Greve, D. N., Treadway, M. T., McGarvey, M., Quinn, B. T., Dusek, J. A., Benson, H., Rauch, S. L., Moore, C. L. et al. (2005). Meditation experience is associated with increased cortical thickness. *NeuroReport*, 16(17), 1893–1897.

Miller, S., Duncan, B., & Hubble, M. (1997). *Escape from Babel: Toward a unifying language for psychotherapy practice*. New York, NY: WW Norton & Company.

Pare, D. (2011) Foreward. In J. Duvall & L. Béres (Eds.), *Innovations in narrative therapy: Connecting practice, training and research*. New York, NY: WW Norton & Company.

Schon, D. (1983). *The reflective practitioner: How professionals think in action*. New York, NY: Basic Books.

Schore, A. (2003). *Affect regulation and the repair of the self*. New York, NY: W. W. Norton & Company Inc.

Siegel, D. (1999). *The developing mind*. New York, NY: Guilford Press.

Siegel, D. (2007). *The mindful brain*. New York, NY: W. W. Norton & Company Inc.

Siegel, D. (2010). *The mindful therapist*. New York, NY: W. W. Norton & Company Inc.

Siegel, S. (2009). *Mindsight*. New York, NY: Random House.

White, M. (1995). *Re-authoring lives: Interviews and essays*. Adelaide, Australia: Dulwich Centre Publications.

White, M. (2007). *Maps of narrative practice*. New York, NY: W. W. Norton & Company Inc.

White, M., & Epston, D. (1990). *Narrative means to therapeutic ends*. New York, NY: W. W. Norton & Company Inc.

Section I

Energizing Clinical Practices with Intriguing and Cutting-Edge Ideas

1 Pivotal Moments, Therapeutic Conversations, and Neurobiology

Landscapes of Resonance, Possibility, and Purpose

Jim Duvall and Robert Maclennan

Introduction

Pivotal moments, "aha" experiences, are natural phenomena that occur in the present moments of everyday life and in therapeutic conversations. As Daniel Stern stated, "[t]he only time of raw subjective reality, of phenomenal experience, is the present moment" (2004, p. 3). Michael White described these moments as epiphanies that "are in harmony with what is precious to people, that's beautiful, that they want to rush toward. . . . What makes them stick is how they are responded to in the outside world" (Duvall & Young, 2009). Pivotal moments make it possible for people to experience an enriched sense of connection with their hopes, and a renewed sense of intimacy with themselves and others (Duvall & Béres, 2011). Pivotal moments are powerful entryways to alternative personal storylines, which open up space for creativity, choice, and connection.

In this chapter we explore the intersection of pivotal moments and brain activity in narrative therapy. This collaborative therapy is situated in postmodern theory, which acknowledges the multiplicity of identities and realities available to people. We offer the analogy of a three-act play, which conceptualizes a therapy session as a story. Focusing on the dominant dispositions of the cerebral hemispheres, we review salient functions of the "social brain" in an attempt to identify and understand factors that may contribute to the occurrence and sustainability of "aha" experiences. Neuroscience has both validated and contributed to our exploration of pivotal moments, giving us a fuller understanding of the relationship between the left and the right hemispheres. This understanding has influenced our use of language, the types of questions we ask, our use of subjective time (Arstilla & Lloyd, 2014), novelty, imagery, and our overall in-the-moment reflexive therapeutic posture.

A story serves as a temporal map, providing space over time to alleviate the problematic effects of life's distressful transitions on people's experience of identity and agency (Duvall & Béres, 2011). People's difficulties are viewed as their attempts to adjust to these transitions. The interpretation of transitional life-stories as "rites of passage" has been handed down through many cultures and generations (Turner, 1977; van Gennep, 1960; White & Epston, 1990). In contrast to a deductive "problem-solving" approach, an inductive "storied" approach introduces reflective practice and critical thinking into the therapeutic process. Herein lies a significant paradigm shift. A deficit-focused problem-solving approach attempts to categorize people and measure them against a predetermined normative standard. An inductive storied approach invites people to step back and view themselves within their social context and, together with others, recall or acquire the knowledge and skills necessary to manage their transition. Thus, they are not the problem. The problem is contextual and they are in relationship with it.

Historical Development: Practice-Based Evidence

My (JD) first time witnessing a pivotal moment was unintentional. It occurred in October 1995 while a colleague and I were routinely viewing a session behind a one-way mirror. A student therapist, Alan, was interviewing a single woman, Sarah. The session was being recorded for supervision purposes. Alan began with a discussion about Sarah's relationship with the problem. He asked a question that invited her to reflect on her abilities:

Alan: Sarah, I'd like to talk with you away from the problem for a while. That will help me to get to know more about the skills and abilities that you have to bring to bear against this problem. Would you tell me about a time in your life when you felt particularly confident about your abilities to handle life's challenges?

Sarah: (Her face relaxed. She looked up to her left.)

Sarah's eye movement up and to her left suggests that she is accessing visual memory via the right cerebral hemisphere (Bourne, 2006).

Alan: (Waiting for a response.) I'm wondering, Sarah, what are your hopes for this session today?

Sarah: (Shook her head, refocused.) I would like you to tell me what to do to loose these feelings of sadness.

Post-Session Debriefing

Following the session, we played the video recording, frame-by-frame for Sarah and then for Alan, so that they could see her responses to his questions.

Sarah: (Watched the playback tearfully.) He asked me to tell him about a time in my life that I felt confident about myself. Suddenly, I remembered when I was 18 years old, standing in my bedroom. I could see the detail of the dark green and yellow flowered wallpaper. I was more confident then than I ever was in my whole life. That's what I want! I want to regain that confidence that I had then and get my life back.

Jim: What was it like when the therapist asked you the second question, which was, "What are your hopes for the session today?"

Sarah: It felt disjointed and pulled me out of my thoughts. I wanted to stay grounded with my memory. I felt connected to myself for the first time in a long time.

We then played the same videotape segment for the therapist.

Alan: Whoa! I didn't notice Sarah having that experience. I thought she couldn't answer the question, and I was trying to ask her a more useful question.

Jim: Now that you do notice her experience, what would you do differently?

Alan: I would slow down and leave space for her to stay with her thoughts. Then, I might say, "It looks like something may have just happened with you. Would it be useful to talk about it, or is it something that's private and you would prefer to keep it to yourself?" I would pay more attention to her responses and manage my responses to her. (Alan voices his intention to develop more "reflexivity," more awareness of his effect on Sarah.)

At that time, we assumed that the pivotal moment experienced by Sarah was an anomaly. Nevertheless, her experience captured our curiosity about the potential contribution of such experiences to person-generated change. We studied the phenomena of pivotal moments further. Our team spent countless hours combing through videotapes and watching numerous live sessions. We discovered that, given the right conditions, pivotal moments were actually commonplace and had been hidden in full view (Stern, 2004)! We wanted to authenticate these transformative thoughts and memories in the moment, to give them "stickability" (Duvall & Béres, 2011, p. 126; Duvall & Young, 2009, p. 18) in the external world. We co-created therapeutic environments that were favorable to the occurrence of pivotal moments, and we trained ourselves to recognize and respond to them as they were occurring.

Neuroscience Makes an Entrance

My (RM) curiosity about pivotal moments developed into a quest to link such epiphanies in therapy with recent discoveries in neuroscience (Maclennan, 2015). Ian McGilchrist (2009) speaks directly to this topic.

He attributes the emergence of "aha" experiences primarily to the activity of the brain's right hemisphere, noting that "this process is not a gradual putting together of bits of information, but an 'aha!' phenomenon—it comes all at once" (p. 47). The right hemisphere, in addition to realizing things suddenly in a flash, also "sees things whole, and in their context" (p. 27); mediates "insight . . . the sort of problem solving that happens when we are . . . not concentrating on it" (p. 65); can "hold several ambiguous possibilities in suspension together without premature closure on the outcome" (p. 72); "with its greater integrative power, is constantly searching for patterns in things" (p. 46); and enables "the appreciation of time, in the sense of something lived through, with a past, present and future" (76). Conceivably, Sarah's experience of transport to her 18-year-old confident self emerged from her intuitive right hemisphere. Realizing this, I became excited by the possibility that neurobiology might help to explain, and even predict, the occurrence and sustainability of "aha" experiences in collaborative therapy.

Although this chapter focuses mainly on the reciprocal functioning of the left and right hemispheres in the co-creation of pivotal moments, the hemispheres represent only the most recent neuronal evolution. All regions of the "triune brain"—the neocortex, the limbic system, and the brainstem—function optimally as an integrated whole. The right hemisphere is more densely interconnected with the bodily nervous system and oriented toward emotion and sensory experience, or "inwardly engaged" life. The left hemisphere is more densely interconnected within itself and oriented toward language and social interaction, or "outwardly engaged" life (Cozolino, 2014; Schore, 2012; Siegel, 2012). Mental functioning involves extensive neocortical and subcortical interaction, including the entire brain and nervous system, with implications considerably beyond the laterality of the hemispheres (Panksepp & Biven, 2012). Together, we recognize that neuroscientific theories can be challenged by new discoveries. Although the consilience of psychotherapy and neurobiology offer much hope and possibility, our proposals are speculative and embedded in an evolving social and scientific context.

Storied Therapy as a Three-Act Play

*Act 1: Separating from Known and Familiar Understandings:
Setting the Stage for Pivotal Moments*

When people arrive at their first therapy session, it's reasonable to assume that they may not be at their best and may even be at their worst. They are likely making "thin" conclusions about themselves or others, thinking, "I'm the problem, or he or she is the problem. My son is ADHD, or my husband is depressed, or I have an anxiety disorder." Immediately, the therapist asks questions that begin to deconstruct and externalize problem-saturated stories. She introduces novelty, ignites curiosity, invites interest, and increases relational engagement. There is an increased appreciation for the complexity of experience and the significance of people's local knowledge. In Act 1, the therapist acts as a conversational manager, assuming a welcoming and participatory posture. She works with people through a partnership, using "co" prefixes (e.g., co-author, co-develop, and co-construct). She invites people to choose what's most important to talk about as they move the story forward.

This inductive conversation, grounded in invitational questions, is competency focused rather than pathology focused. Instead of merely gathering information, the conversation remains *in*-formation and generates experience through a dialogic toing-and-froing between the therapist and the people who consult her. What the therapist hears and perceives is a result of how she participates with others in the conversation. Distance is created from taken-for-granted understandings as they disembark from familiar territory and "perhaps from some status, aspect of identity, or role that is considered to be no longer viable for the person concerned" (White & Epston, 1990, p. 7).

GETTING THE ACT TOGETHER

When people are living under the influence of a problem, their cerebral hemispheres may be functioning at a diminished level of integration. Problem-saturated stories may be tenaciously linked, occluding or excluding other possibility-rich stories. A collaborative therapeutic conversation can help to make visible the subordinated aspects of the larger life-context, linking them together to form alternative storylines. In this creative process of differentiation and association, the participants can embark on a journey toward greater neural, personal, and interpersonal integration (Siegel, 2012).

Briefly above, we outlined the right hemisphere's disposition toward contextual experience and intuitive problem-solving. By contrast, the conceptual, analyzing left hemisphere "sees things abstracted from context, and broken into parts" (McGilchrist, 2009, p. 27); "takes the single solution that seems best to fit what it already knows" (p. 41); "makes up a story, and, lacking insight, appears completely convinced by it" (81); has a "stickiness," a "tendency to recur to what it is familiar with" (p. 86); and "is more concerned with categories and types" (52). When the left hemisphere is "stuck" in a fabricated problem story, it then "re-presents" that story to the right hemisphere, which may "totalize" it, generating problematical moods. In response, the therapist can enlist the instrumental tendency of the left hemisphere, which "is always engaged in a *purpose*" (McGilchrist, 2009, p. 174, italics in original), to construct an interpersonal environment favorable to the experience of pivotal moments (Giorgi, 2011).

A calm, welcoming, regulated, and resonant approach, what Michael White termed a "cool engagement" (White, 2007), can help to activate the body's "social engagement system" to stabilize a person's emotional state. The ventral vagal nerve, a myelinated branch of the parasympathetic nervous system connecting the right side of the brain and major bodily organs, functions to modulate both hyper- and hypo-arousal and enable constructive social interaction (Porges, 2011). Proceeding slowly, waiting for responses, managing ambiguity, and inviting the person "away from the problem" toward preferred experiences can encourage a relaxed reflective state (Duvall & Béres, 2011). And relaxation "favours creativity because it permits broadening of attention, and . . . engagement of the right hemisphere" (McGilchrist, 2009, p. 41). When Alan asked Sarah's permission and inquired about "a time in your life when you felt particularly confident about yourself and your abilities," a pivotal moment ensued. By helping to co-create an empathic and engaged social connection, the therapist can encourage relaxation of the nervous system, activation of the right hemisphere, and the possibility of personal discovery.

ACKNOWLEDGING AND UNPACKING A PIVOTAL MOMENT

People seeking consultation and their therapist often feel energized and changed by pivotal moments. Such experiences are intense, momentous, indeterminate, unrepeatable, and situated in a temporal openness (Bakhtin, 1981; Morson, 1994). As therapists acknowledge these experiences, expressing curiosity and asking questions to "thicken" their meaning, the persons in consultation become engaged and transported. Sarah's memory of her 18-year-old strong and confident self had called into question her assumptions about how she experienced herself in her present life. During such a shift in perspective, change becomes possible. Alan was able to reorient their next conversation to that previous moment of transport.

Alan: Sarah, my understanding is that you were drawn to a memory that left you with a strong emotional experience in our last session. Would it be useful to explore that experience or would you prefer to discuss something else?

Sarah: Yes, I'd like to explore it. I realized that I have already been the person I want to be. When I was 18, I was focused with good friends, plans, and dreams.

Alan: You realized that you have already been who you want to be. I'm curious: What's it like for you to realize this, getting in touch with your former self in this way?

Sarah: When I first came to our last session, I was feeling hopeless. My arms and legs felt like lead. I was feeling very sad.

Alan: (Naming the problem.) So, when you first came for the last ses-
         sion you were feeling hopeless, you felt physically heavy, and you
         were sad. If you could put one word to name these experiences,
         what word would best fit? I'd like you to take your time.

Sarah: (Slowly.) I would call it being in a major rut. I would name it Rut.

Alan: So, when you came to the last session, you were under the influ-
         ence of the Rut. I'm wondering if, over time, the Rut tricked you
         into thinking certain things about yourself, limiting constructive
         possibilities.

Sarah: I wasn't really aware that my life was under the influence of such
         a Rut. When you asked me to remember a time in my life when
         I felt more confident and able to handle life's challenges, all at
         once I had a strong memory of myself when I was 18 years old.
         Zap! I was there, standing in my bedroom. Then I started to
         remember more things from that time, like my friends and the
         things we would do and say together. I felt a really strong sense
         of energy and I wanted to stay there.

When people feel positively engaged, the therapist may invite them
to revisit the problem, naming it and characterizing "negative" features
of it, while deconstructing social constraints. After acknowledging the
"hopelessness" and "sadness," Alan invites Sarah to name her experience. This externalizing practice, "name it to tame it," helps to disarm
the body's fear system and preclude its mobilizing to defend against the
embarrassment of revealing, or the apprehension of reliving, distressing
experiences. Naming stimulates the release of soothing neurotransmit-
ters that calm the limbic amygdala, modulating the fight, flight, or freeze
response (Creswell, Way, Eisenberger, & Lieberman, 2007; Siegel, 2014).
The resulting positive emotions and sense of relief can enlist the right
hemisphere's disposition toward novelty and insight, opening space for
a pivotal experience (Beaudoin, 2015; Kounios & Beeman, 2009; Subramaniam, Kounios, Parrish, & Jung-Beeman, 2008).

After Sarah characterizes her experience as being in a Rut, Alan suggests that the Rut may have "tricked" her. Such characterization may
activate the left hemisphere's analyzing power to define the problem
and, possibly, its competitive streak to resist the problem. In addition,
metaphors like "Rut" and "trick," blending language and image, can
serve to link the left hemisphere's semantic disposition with the right
hemisphere's imaginative capacity. Recalling the moment of transport back to her 18-year-old self, Sarah says, "Zap, I was there. I felt
a strong sense of energy." This sudden, powerful experience emerging
from autobiographical memory illustrates the right hemisphere's preference for "real scenes and stimuli . . . whatever it is that has meaning and
value for us as human beings" (McGilchrist, 2009, p. 56). It is also "the
right hemisphere which gives emotional value to what is seen" (p. 62).

The immediacy and excitement of Sarah's experience suggest an increase in the flow of both information and energy, an indication of enhanced neural integration (Siegel, 2012).

Act 2: Embarking on the Journey: The Landscape of Betwixt and Between

Now, we embark on the journey, the quest, and the *raison d'être* of the therapeutic process. Rich story development is a key feature of this transitional phase, and fertile territory for pivotal moments. Established preoccupation with certainty gives way to an appreciation for the tentativeness of dialogue. This "betwixt and between" phase introduces mystery and possibilities yet unknown. The therapist's responsibility is to facilitate a scaffolding process that supports steady movement across this ambiguous gap, providing a platform for incremental knowledge development.

Pivotal moments arrive partially formed. They are fleeting experiences, vulnerable to disappearance unless they are acknowledged and anchored in the external world. They provide a calling, inviting movement toward a reconsideration and reincorporation of identity. They offer a foundation for people to relate more closely to others, as they often harken back to highly resonant times and places that are inhabited by significant others. They are non-traditional narratives that have grown by association. They are not a task that someone performs with focused logical intent and are more likely to occur when the person is not concentrating on anything. They are expressions of people's internal experiences and memories, what William James called the language of the inner life and *stream of consciousness*: "Where is it, this present? It has melted in our grasp, fled ere we could touch it, gone in the instant of becoming" (James, 1981). Observing a pivotal moment is like witnessing a cinder floating out of a fire pit and disappearing into thin air (Delueze, 1994).

SCENES OF REMEMBERING AND RECONNECTING

Like fish that cannot see the water, people become unwittingly trapped in invisible and pervasive dominant discourses, subjugated to the gripping effects of master narratives (Duvall & Béres, 2011, p. 69). Pivotal moments are powerful experiences that can propel people out of the nullifying effects of everyday life to resonant places and times that support creativity, choice, and a robust sense of self. There are always times when the problem either has less influence, or isn't present. Like panning for gold: traces of preferred stories of identity are always present in these pivotal moments.

A DOUBLE-STORIED ACCOUNT OF SARAH'S IDENTITY

Alan: Sarah, what difference did it make to have your friends close around you?

Sarah: Well, although we spent a lot of time talking about what we were going to do in the future, we were more connected to life through living in the moment.

Alan: Sarah, if feeling hopeless, physically heavy, and sad is called the Rut, then what word would you chose for living in the moment, being more connected to life and having plans for the future? Again, please take your time.

Sarah: Well, I guess I would call that the Groove. (Laughs.) We were really in a groove. Now that groove has turned into a rut. When I was a teenager life was an adventure. Now, we're all a bunch of boring ol' fuddy-duddies. Well, actually one of my friends, Tanya, is kinda cool. Hmm, maybe I could give her a call. I used to ride my bike quite a bit a few years ago. Maybe we could go for a ride together. That would be one step toward being more how I used to be.

Alan: Sarah, would you say that, when you were connected with the Groove, you were an adventurous person?

Sarah: Hmm, that's interesting. I used to be really adventurous and loved to explore new things. I'm calling Tanya. Maybe there's hope.

Previously, Sarah described her life as being in a Rut, stuck in the known and familiar. Alan influenced the conversation toward discovering what is currently unknown and novel and may be possible to know—the "absent but implicit" (Carey, this volume; Carey, Walther, & Russell, 2009; Duvall & Béres, 2011). He invites Sarah to identify what may be "different" about her newly realized preference to be "more connected to life," and he suggests, "take your time." In doing so, he may be addressing a right hemisphere tendency to favor currently implicit (but potentially explicit) aspects of experience—autobiographical memory, unique and unfamiliar associations, and subjective Kairos time as distinct from sequential Cronos time. Sarah then describes her experience of being in the Groove. Recently, neuroscience has discovered that emotional memory is not indelible, but may be changed by experientially activating the problem memory and, within a five-hour "window of activation," repeatedly disconfirming it with a hopeful memory. By juxtaposing experience-near descriptions of the "Rut" and the "Groove," Sarah may be engendering a process of modified "memory reconsolidation" (Ecker, Ticic, & Hulley, 2012; Nader, 2012; Nader and Hardt, 2009).

Alan's careful attuning to Sarah's affective responses, and Sarah's subsequent remembering of her "cool" friend, implies an increasing mutual engagement of the social brain. Collaborative therapy and neuroscience suggest that we learn who we are through social interaction. This capacity for resonance and empathy—aspects of theory of mind—involves neuronal activation in the "observer" mirroring neuronal activation in the "actor," especially when the action involves intention (Decety & Lamm, 2006; Decety & Meyer, 2008; Rizzolatti, Fadiga, Fogassi, & Gallese, 1999). Theory of mind is mediated by "mirror neurons" interconnecting many regions of the brain (Cozolino, 2014). And the emotional aspect of social understanding, "in the sense of empathic connection, as well as understanding how others feel . . . is made possible by the right hemisphere" (McGilchrist, 2009, p. 66). Empathy enables Alan to appreciate Sarah's emotional involvement, and allows Sarah to share her friend's personal enthusiasms. Resonating with, and being mirrored by, another person can be a profoundly integrating experience.

In confirmation of Alan's apparent resonance with her evolving story, Sarah asserts, "I'm going forward to re-discover my confident and adventurous self!" While mirroring of the external environment involves more lateralized regions of the brain, involvement with the internal environment, or sense of self, is mediated primarily by midline cortical and subcortical structures. In response to her novel pivotal discoveries, Sarah is experiencing a revived energy, personal agency, and sense of self. A relative absence of external stimuli facilitates such self-focus. "Stimulus-independent thought . . . allows us to internalize and manipulate images, play out interpersonal scenarios, and process emotions. . . . in imaginal space within the flow of time" (Cozolino, 2014, p. 377. Also Northoff & Bermpohl, 2004; Northoff et al. 2006). Collaboratively reclaiming and reconnecting with formerly eclipsed but currently preferred memories and experiences, values, and relationships helps to fortify the sense of self, activate multiple regions of the triune brain, and enhance movement toward neural and personal integration.

CO-CONSTRUCTING A REFLECTING SURFACE

Implicit learnings that arise from pivotal moments during the transitional phase can be strung together to form alternative storylines, which can be contrasted with the oppressive dominant storyline that people bring to the therapeutic process. Throughout the session, as illustrated in the previous transcript, the therapist offers reflecting summaries at regular intervals, paraphrasing key words and phrases, and receiving both verbal and non-verbal verification from the person seeking consultation, ensuring that they remain in sync with one another. This inductive posture invites people to reflect in and on the conversation, make discernments about their lives, and illuminate gaps between the influences of the problem story and their strongly held values. The reflecting summary that creates the threshold to Act 3 summarizes the entire therapeutic conversation and reaches back in time to the pre-problem past, integrating prior values and skills with new learnings.

This comprehensive reflecting summary, weaving preferred values and hopeful memories into the problem story, may supplement the fabricating function of the left hemisphere and "re-present" previously implicit, but now explicit, experience back to the right hemisphere, for integration into the life-story. This new narrative—by combining the sequential, logical, semantic capacity of the left hemisphere with the holistic, emotional, episodic memory of the right hemisphere—can be a powerful agent of neural, personal, and interpersonal integration (Cozolino, 2014; Siegel, 2012).

Act 3: The Reincorporation of Identity

New learnings that were acquired from pivotal moments that occurred in Act 2 are now integrated with skills and abilities that existed in the pre-problem past, to encourage a reincorporation of identity (Turner, 1977; van Gennep, 1960; White & Epston, 1990). This reincorporation can be experienced when people imagine being in "another place," leaving behind an aspect of identity that is no longer required, while being in touch with a preferred sense of self.

Conclusion

The focus of this chapter has been the illumination of pivotal moments. We described, through the analogy of the storied approach of the three-act-play, how merging the concepts and practices of collaborative therapy with recent discoveries from neuroscience can produce a consilience, in which two independent and seemingly unrelated disciplines converge to produce robust results. The benefits of this consilience are substantial, and challenge many taken-for-granted ideas and practices. With reference to brain function, especially the relative dispositions of the cerebral hemispheres, we suggested that collaborative therapy might be regarded as a process of differentiation, association, and integration on neural, personal, and interpersonal levels.

References

Arstila, V. & Lloyd, D. (Eds.) (2014) *Subjective time: The philosophy, psychology, and neuroscience of temporality.* Cambridge, MA. The MIT Press.

Bakhtin, M. (1981). *The dialogic imagination: Four essays* (Ed. Michael Holquist. Trans. Caryl Emerson & Michael Holquist). Austin and London: University of Texas Press.

Beaudoin, M.-N. (2015). Flourishing with positive emotions: Increasing clients' repertoire of problem counter-states. *Journal of Systemic Therapies*, 3(34), 1–13.

Bourne, V. J. (2006). The divided visual field paradigm: Methodological considerations. *Laterality, 11*, 373–393.

Carey, M., Walther, S., & Russell, S. (2009). The absent but implicit: A map to support therapeutic enquiry. *Family Process, 48*(3), 319–331.

Cozolino, L. (2014). *The neuroscience of human relationships: Attachment and the developing social brain* (2nd ed.). New York, NY: W. W. Norton & Company Inc.

Creswell, J., Way, B., Eisenberger, N., & Lieberman, M. (2007). Neural correlates of dispositional mindfulness during affect labeling. *Psychosomatic Medicine, 69*, 560–565.

Decety, J., & Lamm, C. (2006). Human empathy through the lens of social neuroscience. *The Scientific World Journal, 6*, 1146–1163.

Decety, J., & Meyer, M. (2008). From emotional resonance to empathic understanding: A social developmental neuroscience account. *Development and Psychopathology, 20*, 1053–1080.

Delueze, G. (1994). *Difference and repetition*. New York, NY: Columbia University Press. (Original work published in 1968, Presse Universitaires de France, in French).

Duvall, J., & Béres, L. (2011). *Innovations in narrative therapy: Connecting practice training and research*. New York, NY: W. W. Norton & Company Inc.

Duvall, J., & Young, K. (2009). Keeping faith: A conversation with Michael White. *Journal of Systemic Therapies, 28*(1), 1–18.

Ecker, B., Ticic, R., & Hulley, L. (2012). *Unlocking the emotional brain: Eliminating symptoms at their roots using memory reconsolidation*. New York, NY: Routledge.

Giorgi, B. (2011). A phenomenological analysis of the experience of pivotal moments in therapy as defined by clients. *Journal of Phenomenological Psychology, 42*, 61–106.

James, W. (1981). *The principles of psychology*. Cambridge, MA: Harvard University Press.

Kounios, J., & Beeman, M. (2009). The aha! moment: The cognitive neuroscience of insight. *Current Directions in Psychological Science, 18*(4), 210–216.

Maclennan, R. (2015). Co-creating pivotal moments: Narrative practice and neuroscience. *Journal of Systemic Therapies, 34*(1), 43–60.

McGilchrist, I. (2009). *The master and his emissary: The divided brain and the making of the Western world*. New Haven, CT: Yale University Press.

Morson, G. (1994). *Narrative and freedom: The shadows of time*. New Haven, CT: Yale University Press.

Nader, K. (2012). *Memory manipulation*. Retrieved from https://www.youtube.com/watch?v+Dan68pTqpxQ

Nader, K., & Hardt, O. (2009). A single standard for memory: The case for reconsolidation. *Nature Reviews Neuroscience, 10*, 224–234.

Northoff, G., & Bermpohl, F. (2004). Cortical midline structures and the self. *Trends in Cognitive Science, 3*(8), 102–107.

Northoff, G., Heinzel, A., de Greck, M., Bermpohl, F., Dobrowolny, H., & Panksepp, J. (2006). Self-referential processing in our brain: A meta-analysis of imaging studies on the self. *NeuroImage, 31*, 440–457.

Panksepp, J., & Biven, L. (2012). *The archeology of mind: Neuroevolutionary origins of human emotions*. New York, NY: Norton.

Porges, S. (2011). *The polyvagal theory: Neurophysiological foundations of emotions, attachment, communication, and self-regulation.* New York, NY: W. W. Norton & Company Inc.

Rizzolatti, G., Fadiga, L., Fogassi, L., & Gallese, V. (1999). Resonance behaviors and mirror neurons. *Archives Italiennes de Biologie, 137,* 85–100.

Schore, A. (2012). *The science of the ART of psychotherapy.* New York, NY: W. W. Norton & Company Inc.

Siegel, D. (2012). *The developing mind: How relationships and the brain interact to shape who we are* (2nd ed.). New York, NY: Guilford Press.

Siegel, D. (2014). *Name it to tame it.* Dalai Lama Centre for Peace and Education. Retrieved from https://www.youtube.com/watch?v=ZcDLzppD4Jc

Stern, D. (2004). *The present moment in psychotherapy and everyday life.* New York, NY: W. W. Norton & Company Inc.

Subramaniam, K., Kounios, J., Parrish, T. B., & Jung-Beeman, M. (2008). A brain mechanism for facilitation of insight by positive affect. *Journal of Cognitive Neuroscience, 21*(3), 415–432.

Turner, V. (1977). *The ritual process: Structure and anti-structure.* Ithaca, NY: Cornell University Press. (Original work published in 1969).

van Gennep, A. (1960). *The rites of passage.* Chicago: University of Chicago Press. (Original work published in 1909).

White, M. (2007). *Maps of narrative practices.* New York, NY: W. W. Norton & Company Inc.

White, M., & Epston, D. (1990). *Narrative means to therapeutic ends.* New York, NY: W. W. Norton & Company Inc.

2 Helping Clients Thrive with Positive Emotions[1]

Expanding People's Repertoire of Problem Counter-States

Marie-Nathalie Beaudoin

A large number of clients come to therapy because they are distressed and feel unable to contain the intensity of their affective experience. For example, some clients may report being fully aware that they should not be so anxious or stressed about the small obstacles of life but are still captured affectively regardless of their best intentions and well-developed alternative ways of being. Others may feel annoyed with themselves for being overly sensitive in relationship but struggle with inhibiting the easily triggered flood of hurtful feelings even if they understand its origin and meaning. Across theoretical orientations, there are reports of clients who struggle with physiologically engrained feelings that override their rational cognitive processes in spite of their best efforts, intentions, and re-authoring journey. A closer look at recent work in neuro-affective sciences will provide a better understanding of this situation and open doors to new practices which can allow therapists to better help these clients.

Relevant Neuro-Affective Studies

Since the discovery that intense emotions can "override" the brain's cognitive processes (Damasio, 2000; LeDoux, 2000, 2002), scientists have become increasingly interested in examining the neurological activation patterns associated with people's affective experiences. Specific emotions do not seem to have consistent patterns of activation in the brain across individuals, ages, intensity, and cultures (Panksepp & Biven, 2012). Affect, however, based on its dichotomous classification of feelings based on their positive or negative valence, has been found to be associated with more consistent patterns of activation. Affect has been defined as the "experience of feeling" and is characterized on a neurological level by three markers: arousal (impulsion to act), intensity (activation of the nervous system), and valence (positive or negative). More specifically, affect typically experienced as "negative" tends to activate specific limbic areas of the brain involved in the fight, flight, freeze, faint system. On the other hand, affective states falling in the "positive" categories are associated with various patterns of left hemisphere activation (Lindquist, Wager,

Kober, Bliss-Moreau, & Barrett, 2012). The effects of negative versus positive emotions on the brain will now be reviewed in more detail.

Negative affect reduces the blood flow to the frontal lobe, diminishes the ability to connect, reduces attention to peripheral information, narrows attention, increases the production of cortisol (stress hormone), and engages the fight, flight, or freeze system (Siegel, 2012). Negative affect also shapes the brain in powerful ways both at the structural and cellular level. For example, research has shown that, on average, sadness can activate up to 35 regions of the brain, anger 13, and fear 11 (Vytal & Hamann, 2010). In contrast happiness seems to activate only an average of nine regions. At the cellular level, neural networks triggered frequently tend to become faster (more myelin and dendrites) and interconnected in a pattern of response that has an increasing probability of being triggered with every activating event (Siegel, 2010, 2012). For example, each time a person reacts with intense fear, this response's neural connection in the brain becomes slightly stronger, faster, and more likely to be activated in the next similar event. Therapists are therefore swimming upstream when it comes to moving away from problem-dominated affective experiences and boosting clients' preferred selves. Intense negative-affect-related problems such as depression, which have been recurring over a long period of time, can become difficult to address and recur more easily.

Positive affect, in contrast, is not triggered as easily and intensely, but is associated with increased mental capacities, health, and wellbeing. More specifically, positive affect is associated with higher levels of attention and cognitions, a greater repertoire of considered actions, increased intrinsic motivation and openness to trying new things, enhanced critical thinking, perspective taking, better impulse control, and increased likelihood of finding meaning. A study of 188 participants recording daily accounts of their affective experiences over 28 days found that individuals who flourish and are most successful in their lives tend to live a ratio of three positive moments for each negative one (Fredrickson & Losada, 2005). Positive affect benefits from being encouraged since most people tend to spend the majority of their time dwelling in neutral or negative states. In the neurobiology literature, this is explained by the brain's natural bias to pay attention to events that may threaten survival, which has led some authors to describe the brain as being "like Velcro for negative emotions" (Hansen, 2013). Some of this phenomenon can also be understood as a socio-cultural failure to encourage the noticing and embracing of more subtle moments of satisfaction in life. In the end, even when living an experience that could be positive, a lot of well-functioning people forget to fully enjoy a satisfying moment. This lack of attention to satisfying moments can be even more engrained in clients who have struggled with problems for a long time. Many have progressively been mentally and emotionally captured by dominant problem stories, or cognitive or affective biases, to notice only problem-confirming events.

Affect in Therapy

Most therapists, regardless of theoretical orientation, are trained to help clients overcome problematic experiences. Therapy is usually terminated when clients have found a certain level of peace with their problems, changed their behaviors or context of life, or revisited their views of themselves, their relationships, or the situation. For example, a client struggling with self-doubt may be assisted in finding self-confidence; a client with impulse control issues will have developed ways of containing strong urges; a client with anxiety may have connected with an ability to be calmer. Therapists often assume that clients are now "free" to be happy. While some clients may indeed shift to a satisfying existence, others remain relatively disconnected from positive affect after having spent so much time in a negative space.

Flourishing with positive affect involves emotions such as joy, appreciation, gratitude, love, care, and satisfaction, which are different states than common therapeutic outcomes such as feeling calm, self-confident, resilient, accepting, patient or self-forgiving, to name only a few. The ability to notice the little gifts of life, and connect with small moments of positive emotions, increases the likelihood of experiencing happiness and flourishing. Adding positive affect and emotions to therapeutic journeys offers three main benefits: new valuable memories, additional problem counter-states, and emotional intensity. Each of these benefits will now be discussed in more depth.

First, clients given an opportunity to enrich their preferred experiences of themselves with positive affect often reconnect with a collection of new memories not previously included in their re-authoring. This mainly occurs because of the well-known mood congruent recall phenomena (also called state dependent recall) where the brain tends to more readily remember events previously encoded in similar emotional states. Associating a positive affect with the preferred experience of oneself strengthens its associated neural network, and expands its connections to a greater number of life experiences. For example, Donna, age 24, was very worried about her sister's health issues. While the health issues were in no way life threatening, the "Worries" got Donna to imagine the death and funeral of her sister. These images were very distressing since the two sisters were close in age and had always enjoyed a rewarding sibling relationship. A number of externalizing conversations (White, 2007) helped Donna regain control of the "Worries," and a "Calm and Supportive" preferred self was developed. Donna did not want to distress or burden her sister with her own emotional struggles. When asked which positive emotion could emerge out of a calm and supportive interaction with her sister, Donna paused and then exclaimed: "humor!" When prompted to explain, she recalled a brief moment when her sister had been referred for an MRI and she had connected with the calm state explored in therapy, and then shifted to playfully teasing her using old family stories. Once humor was identified, therapeutic conversations could then expand on this rich alternative way of being and the multiple satisfying experiences associated with it. The embodied sensations associated with calm and humor were also explored in detail so the client could more readily access those states. The preferred self of being humorous may have emerged otherwise but not necessarily. With this particular client, it probably wouldn't have spontaneously arisen given the worrisome atmosphere of her sister facing complex medical problems. Prompting directly and actively for positive experiences was helpful to this client.

Second, clients may have been struggling to control a distressing emotional experience for a long time and have developed ways to partially handle the problem without being able to significantly reduce its chronic grip on their lives. Exploring a positive emotion that could counter the problematic state offers a second option from which to contain or eradicate the problem. For example, a therapist had been struggling with nervousness for a long time and volunteered to be interviewed, live, in one of the author's workshops. This nervousness particularly arose in the context of professional settings when the interviewee herself was teaching. While the interviewee had developed a number of helpful mindfulness practices to ground herself before teaching, and had explored a preferred self of being calm, she was annoyed by the fact that she still had to face this problem every time and could only manage to limit its intensity. When invited to connect the preferred self of calm with a positive emotion, she readily came up with: "Joy." She then explained that the process of expanding beyond being calm and into a positive state led her to suddenly notice more aspects of her personal and professional life that she cherished. This joy broadened and shifted her appraisal of her experience, which was in sharp contrast with the narrower, internally focused, self-deprecating effects of nervousness. Joy could also match and even surpass the intensity and vividness of nervousness whereas calm couldn't. The interviewee left the conversation feeling that she now had two options to handle the nervousness: she could choose to either connect with experiences of oneself as calm (the previously identified preferred self) or tap into the affective counter-state of joyfulness (the newly recognized alternative experience of herself).

Third, positive emotions may be associated with more intense or distinct sets of physiological manifestations for some clients. Well-known, desirable positive emotions may be easier to tap into than a preferred state such as self-confidence, for example, which may feel newer, blurry, and harder to physiologically enter. The more familiar and "viscerally" felt the emotional experience, the greater the likelihood that a client can intentionally reconnect with the state as a viable step away from the problem. For example, when prompted to associate a positive emotion with a "determined" preferred self, a middle-aged man, Raphael, reconnected with the feeling of pride that was completely obscured by the problem of depression. Tapping in the emotional state of pride reminded Raphael of specific moments and important people not recalled when simply exploring "determination," even if they were indirectly relevant and therefore enriching of re-storying. A positive emotion, especially when explored in embodied ways, can therefore act as a more clearly delineated counter-state to the problem, or as a transitional experience between the problem experience and the chosen preferred self.

Three Specific Clinical Practices to Boost Positive Affect

Since problems and distressing emotions have a physiological component (often affecting the face, shoulders, posture, breath, heart rate, etc.), preferred selves and experiments with positive emotions also benefit from being felt and described in embodied ways (Beaudoin & Zimmerman, 2011). All of the practices below benefit from this enrichment.

(a) **Positive Affect during Therapeutic Conversations: Expanding and Uplifting**

The exploration of satisfying experiences of oneself can be initiated at the beginning of the therapeutic process (Epston, 2010) or after hearing clients' accounts of problems. In either case, clients can be invited to connect to positive experiences of themselves after having lingered in a preferred self or richly explored a moment handled in a satisfying way. From a scaffolding standpoint, it is easier for clients to take a step in the direction of positive affect when they've just been discussing a meaningful effort, moment, or success (unique outcome). The easiest question to ask to initiate this process is: "If this experience of letting go was to be connected to a positive emotion, what would it be?" This question usually requires a few seconds of thinking but is invariably answered with intrigue and enthusiasm, as it opens the door to a new world of stories, events, relationships, people, places, and times that can be explored. This fresh territory of discussion is freeing as it is no longer directly in opposition to, and therefore limited by, its position against the problem.

(b) **Encoding Positive Affect Right after the Session: Dwelling Fosters Strengthening**

As we know, effective therapeutic conversations can trigger a shift in clients' experiences of themselves and their lives. From a neurobiological point of view, this shift from a problem view to a viscerally felt preferred experience involves a change in the brain's synaptic firing. More specifically, when old beliefs and experiences are examined in therapy and altered by new perspectives and evocative meanings, there is a progressive change in synaptic connections which is reflected in subsequent memory storage. The brain's re-encoding of experience infused with new material involves "memory re-consolidation." Memory re-consolidation has been found to take approximately five hours during which the experience to be stored can remain particularly malleable (Nader & Einarsson, 2010). Since therapeutic conversations typically last about an hour (after which clients often go back to a context of life that may support the problem), how can we increase the likelihood that preferred experiences brought forth in therapy will better endure throughout the consolidation period? One way is to invite clients to dwell in the positive state while leaving the therapist's office by giving them a small mental task to do as they are driving or walking away. For example, at the end of the session, clients can be given a pad of paper titled "Take-Aways" on which they are encouraged to take notes during the therapist's summarizing of the session. A particular emphasis is given to newfound details on counter-states and positive affect. When relevant, clients are then asked to remember other life events associated with this specific positive emotion or preferred self, and instructed to add to the written document when they get home. If driving away, clients can also be encouraged to listen to music which would sustain the positive emotion, and maybe even increase it. Music has been found to enhance emotions and autobiographical memories (Jancke, 2008). When clients follow these suggestions, it is not uncommon for them to remember new events supporting the material discussed and to spend more of their own time dwelling on helpful memories. Therapists can then begin the following session by touching base on clients' previous post-therapy thoughts and experiences.

(c) **Strengthening Positive Affect between Sessions: Noticing Allows Repeating**

In an effort to further the development of neural networks associated with positive affect, clients can be encouraged to keep track of preferred experiences of self and positive emotions between sessions. Keeping track of one's experiences is increasingly popular in our world saturated with various social media. People have become accustomed to the process of monitoring and posting what they're doing, and how they're feeling, on various websites. With the technological advancement of phones and a large number of available apps, recording a moment of satisfaction is a click away. While the cumulative daily list of observations may offer some interesting insights on preferred selves and positive emotions such as frequency, time of the day, relationships, and contexts, the process itself of being on the lookout for potentially satisfying experiences and positive affect is ultimately of the greatest value. The stance of searching for opportunities for positive emotions can shift a client's focus from one that is problem saturated to one of noticing even small possibilities of well-being. These can be as simple as appreciating a child's smile or the absence of traffic going home. Since people typically find what they are looking for, noticing more opportunities for satisfying moments gives people the impression that they are receiving little gifts from life. This noticing can eventually take on a life of its own, increase the neural encoding of this way of being, and facilitate the repetition of positive experiences of self.

Clinical Example

Rangi is a 65-year-old Indian woman who has lost her husband eight years ago and is struggling with boredom and depressed feelings. She had been a bright and successful Silicon Valley engineer before she and her husband had chosen to retire early to travel. Now on her own, with her two adult children living in another state, she can't seem to find anything enjoyable or stimulating to occupy her time, aside from her occasional hikes with two precious friends (who have jobs and families of their own).

In the first session, Rangi shared that she had moved on from the actual loss of her husband but felt a sense of emptiness as she has nothing to do and no one to keep her company. Therapeutic conversations focused on externalizing the "Emptiness feeling" that captured her experience in a very vivid and visceral way. Amongst other things, this feeling made her feel useless, tired, unmotivated to go out, and refrain from trying new activities, which were assumed to be boring. We also explored how her favorite experience of herself was when she Skyped with her grandchildren, as she felt connected and valued in her contributions to their lives. Given the importance of expanding on this experience, I asked her a number of questions to associate feeling connected with a richer set of positive emotions (practice a). In particular, when asked which positive emotion could arise out of her conversation with her grandchildren, she answered "intrigue" and "joy." She felt intrigued in their developing minds and curious about how they saw the world. She rejoiced in interacting with them in playful ways. Once identified, her embodied experience of these positive emotions was explored in depth to increase her awareness, intensity of these sensations, and neural availability. The more a person dwells in a certain state, the more readily available this state becomes for future neural firing. Rangi felt that these positive emotions triggered a "twinkling" in her heart. I encouraged her to document moments when that feeling was present, and to find something to do right after our session that might fuel the intrigue, joy, and twinkling in her heart (practice b). Rangi is now coming for a follow-up visit.

MN: At the end of our last session, I encouraged you to do something that would build on our conversation. We had talked about expanding on the feelings of "joy" and "intrigue." I wonder what might have stayed with you from that conversation, and if you had the time to try that or not?

When I give clients an assignment, it is always done with the caveat that they can choose to do it or not. I stress that this is a suggestion that I think could be very beneficial but that I won't be offended if they do not follow through. When they come to their subsequent meeting, I make sure to follow up in a way that would elicit the least possible amount of discomfort or embarrassment, if they haven't done the assignment. Rangi however has tried it.

R: Well, since I actually had plenty of time after our session, I decided to stop at the "Move It Elsewhere" store near your office.

MN: Oh! I don't know that store, what kind of store is it?

R: It's an after estate sale. When people pass away, all their unwanted belongings end up there.

MN: Okay, so you stopped at that store. What compelled you to go there after our meeting?

R (smiling): Well, I liked the idea of expanding on our conversation about "joy" and "intrigue," and had always felt a glimmer of intrigue when I drove past this shop but then never wanted to bother with parking.

MN: So you paid attention to feeling "intrigued" and made the decision to stop? (Nods)

Here I am debating between getting more information about the unfolding of the event itself, or exploring the embodied experience of feeling "intrigued" and having acted on it. Since I'm not sure if anything significant evolved from stopping at the store, I decide to get more information before making a choice. Once I have the big picture of the event, I can come back to the moment that seems most meaningful.

MN: What effect did it have on you to bother with parking and try it out?

R: This store is a good reminder that we need to live our life now instead of saving things for a future which may never come. It was an interesting place to visit and I may have discovered a new hobby: Vinyl doll restoration.

MN: Vinyl doll restoration??

R: Yes, this store has many old and damaged dolls that were obviously well loved by some children before. It's sad that no one wants them anymore, they're all dusty. They have a happy "vibe" even if they're damaged. I just bought one to fix it up as a hobby and then realized I could sell it on Ebay for ten times more. I know it's silly but since we had talked about the joy I experience when I contribute to someone or something, I thought I'd try to bring a doll back to life. So I've been spending time doing that.

I am delighted by the unexpected news and considering which direction to go out of the many choices competing in my mind, such as: How did the decision to purchase the doll arise when she was in the store? Was purchasing the doll another effect of intrigue or did it come out of another experience of herself? Did she debate with herself whether to buy or not? What was the winning argument to purchase it? What does the doll look like and does she have a vision for the restoration? Will the new image of the doll remind her of a precious doll she might have loved as a child? Since she left the store, which moment was most exciting or infused with joy? What difference does it make to have tried a new hobby? From this whirlwind of questions in my mind, and based on my interest in neurobiology, positive emotions, and scaffolding, I decide to focus on the following:

MN: What is it like for you to spend time on bringing a doll back to life and restore it, does it bring some joy?

R: It actually does!

MN: Can you tell me more about the joy it brings you?

R: Well, the whole process of making it beautiful again is satisfying but also it feels good to rescue her from a landfill. She can make someone happy again *and* she won't pollute the world.

MN: So there's a double joy, contributing to someone's happiness and not polluting the world? (Nods) Does that connect to some beliefs or values that have some importance for you in your life?

R: Hum . . . Now that we are talking about it, yes, I really value re-using, it's like setting this doll free to live another life and have it bring joy to others. People in my culture really believe in this interconnection. There's something Zen in there for me.

MN: Zen in which way?

R: Well, an object is meaningless in and of itself, what matters is the experience it can give someone. Working on my doll has given me a reason to get out of bed in the morning, and gives value to this doll. This way we both have a helpful role in the world.

MN: Can you tell me more about when you felt this helpful role in the world and were last working on your doll?

R: It was this morning, I was working on her hair and was excited about how it was shaping up, even though this is my first time doing such a thing.

MN: How would you describe the sensation of excitement in your body?

R: The excitement was like some kind of tingling, or like there was warmth and glitter in my throat and chest. I hadn't felt like that in a long time.

MN: If you close your eyes, can you connect with those sensations right now?

R: Yes, I think a lot of it is still with me.

MN: What are you noticing about your body that lets you know it is still with you?

It is valuable to spend time here, exploring sensations and their descriptions. Clients can be invited to sit with those experiences, close their eyes, and breathe deeply while focusing on their inner sensations. This process contributes to fixing those moments to memory in the richest possible way. After doing this for a minute or so, it is helpful to look for other related events supporting positive and preferred emotions. In collaborative therapies, this linking of multiple preferred moments through time reinforces people's preferred identities (re-authoring) and, in neurobiology, the connection of multiple experiences of positive emotions reinforces the associated neural network.

MN: Was that excitement nourished even in small ways by other experiences today?

R: Hum . . . I guess when I went shopping it felt less like a drag, I was looking for stuff for me and her, and was probably nicer with the clerk . . . I noticed kids in their strollers more and the type of dolls or stuffed animals they had with them. I smiled more. And then I had something new to talk with my friends.

The conversation continues with two main therapeutic intentions. First, highlighting different moments when this client connected to joy and intrigue, making this positive experience more salient and richly available in her mind. Second, facilitating an increased awareness of the implications associated with intentionally connecting with this brain state. "People become who they practice to be" (Beaudoin, 2014), and sometimes, choosing consciously to enter in a certain state can activate the neural networks enough to then genuinely experience that preferred state. At the end of our session, I encourage Rangi to write down a preferred experience of herself every day before our next meeting (practice c).

Clients can easily go back to their problem-saturated world and see therapy as a weekly buoy to keep their heads above water. There is a good likelihood that none of this material would have been available had Rangi not been encouraged to build upon the experiences of "joy" and "intrigue" after our session. Invitations to take initiatives to expand on positive therapeutic experiences after sessions can broaden the repertoire of problem counter-states and allows re-authoring to migrate more readily into daily life.

Clinical Limitations

Clinically, the practice of enriching therapeutic conversations with positive affect needs to be introduced carefully, especially with clients struggling with a more negative outlook. If the client is not accessing positive affect during the therapeutic session and has a very problem-saturated life, such practice could feel alienating, disconnected from experience, and even further support the problem with conclusions such as "there are no moments of satisfaction in my life." The observation assignment is helpful if introduced when relevant, at key moments in the therapeutic process, and when clients can benefit from completing it in the context of their lives.

Conclusion

This chapter has offered an overview of the literature on positive affect and its value in therapeutic conversations. Therapists are encouraged to move beyond assisting clients with problems and facilitate a process by which people will flourish and thrive. Benefits of actively exploring positive emotions include tapping into a rich collection of unstoried memories, accessing intense emotions that can more effectively replace problem states, and developing additional options to counteract problem-infused experiences.

Note

1. A portion of this material was presented in the plenary to the Winds of Change conference "Interpersonal Neurobiology and Innovative Therapeutic Practices" on April 24th, 2014, in Toronto, Canada. The theoretical section of this chapter is reprinted with permission (*Journal of Systemic Therapies*, *34(3)*, 1–12, 2015), and includes an expanded clinical section with an unpublished transcript of a conversation with a client.

References

Beaudoin, M.-N. (2014). *Boosting all children's social and emotional brain power: Life transforming activities.* Thousand Oaks, CA: Corwin Press.

Beaudoin, M.-N., & Zimmerman, J. (2011). Narrative therapy and interpersonal neurobiology: Revisiting classic practices, developing new emphases. *Journal of Systemic Therapies*, 48(1), 1–13.

Damasio, A. (2000). *The feeling of what happens: Body and emotions in the making of consciousness.* New York, NY: Mariner.

Epston, D. (2010). The corner: Stories this time. *Journal of Systemic Therapies*, 29(4), 92–102.

Fredrickson, B. L., & Losada, M. F. (2005). Positive affect and the complex dynamics of human flourishing. *American Psychologist*, 60, 678–686.

Hansen, R. (2013). *Hardwiring happiness.* New York, NY: Harmony Books.

Jancke, J. (2008). Music, memory and emotion. *Journal of Biology*, 7(21), 33–43.

LeDoux, J. E. (2000). Emotional circuits in the brain. *Annual Review of Neuroscience*, 23, 155–184.

LeDoux, J. E. (2002). *Synaptic self: How our brains become who we are.* New York, NY: Penguin Books.

Lindquist, K., Wager, T., Kober, H., Bliss-Moreau, E., & Barrett, L. F. (2012). The brain basis of emotion: A meta-analytic review. *Behavioral Brain Sciences*, 35, 121–143.

Nader, K., & Einarsson, E. (2010). Memory reconsolidation: An update. *Annals of the New York Academy of Sciences, 1191*, 27–47.

Panksepp, J., & Biven, L. (2012). *The archeology of mind: Neuroevolutionary origins of human emotions.* New York, NY: W. W. Norton & Company Inc.

Siegel, D. (2010). *The mindful therapist.* New York, NY: W. W. Norton & Company Inc.

Siegel, D. (2012). *The developing mind: How relationships and the brain interact to shape who we are* (2nd ed.). New York, NY: Guilford Press.

Vytal, K., & Hamann, S. (2010). Neuroimaging support for discrete neural correlates of basic emotions: A voxel-based meta-analysis. *Journal of Cognitive Neuroscience, 22*(12), 2864–2885.

White, M. (2007). *Maps of narrative practice.* New York, NY: W. W. Norton & Company Inc.

3 From Implicit Experience to Explicit Stories

Maggie Carey

Alison was not at ease at our first meeting. She had had trouble finding my office, was flustered and found it difficult to relax; as she drank from the glass of water that I offered, her hand shook and water spilled on the table. *"Ah, I shouldn't have come here,"* she said, *"It's all a big mistake. Talking about things has never helped."* She then started to cry and to apologies for the tears, saying, *"You must think I'm stupid. Sometimes I can't stop once I start."* It was clear that Alice's state of agitation was not conducive to a therapeutic enquiry that was aimed at helping her make sense of her experience. Any exploration of what was problematic was most likely to contribute to further distress and upset and could even trigger a panic attack.

There is a lot that is now known about the impact of traumatic stress on neurobiological function, particularly in regard to what happens when we are faced with threat of danger, and also on what memories we are left with of the traumatic experience (LeDoux, 1996). As a response to traumatic events our brains are organized to protect us. Evolving as we did with little natural protection and lacking sharp teeth, strength, and speed, our brains developed with an arrangement that gave us the best possible chance of survival in a dangerous world. As a response to imminent threat, it was not going to be good enough to leave things to the relatively slow processes of the frontal cortex to work out what we should do. We needed an alarm system that could operate without thinking, and that could automatically activate the body functions that we would need to fight, flee or freeze in the face of danger.

In my clinical practice with women and children who have experienced violence and abuse, or the trauma of neglect, I have been drawn to understanding the operations of the neurobiological processes that occur in the face of severe threat to bodily safety or to the psychological or emotional sense of self. My work is grounded in the practice of Narrative Therapy and the understanding that it is through stories that we have a sense of ourselves and that these stories shape how we experience our lives (Russell & Carey, 2004). We are not born with the stories of self that we come to have, but rather they are developed socially and relationally as we go through life and as we make meaning of what we are experiencing. Neurobiologists are increasingly referring to this capacity to develop stories as the way in which our brains function. (Broks, 2004; LeDoux, 1996). Memories are stories through which we selectively link events together over time according to a plot or theme.

Michael White, one of the founders of Narrative Therapy, introduced practices that could support the development of stories that were different from what the story of the trauma was telling the person. The trauma story often constructs an account of the person as being damaged, broken, weak, a victim, and incapable of doing life. These accounts of self serve to limit and curtail the person's belief in their ability to move forward in their lives and often leave them stuck in a 'single' story of being 'victim.' While the memory of the traumatic experience will not be erased through therapy, there are other meanings of what happened that can come to be more influential, and the plastic nature of brain function tells us that it is always possible to develop new stories. There is the story of the trauma and then there is the story of how the person responded to what happened.

These 'double-storied' accounts (White, 2000) are implied by the presence of emotional pain. The presence of pain tells us that there is something that the person gives value to that has been violated or transgressed through the experience of trauma. The pain can be seen as an indication of the person holding certain intentions, principles or understandings of life that have been trodden on. It can also be seen as a refusal to go along with what happened, a refusal to say it didn't matter. The stories that are brought forward in this way can be developed into rich or thick accounts that provide a different experience of 'self' and a different place to stand in relation to what has been traumatic. In developing these new stories, new neural pathways are being developed and having these stories as other places to stand lessens the likelihood of re-traumatization and the triggering of the autonomic nervous system (ANS).

The automatic responses of the ANS are set in motion when we are experiencing threat and danger. They are centered in the older part of our brains, involving the limbic system, which includes the thalamus, the hypothalamus, the amygdala and the hippocampus. The significant aspect of these processes is the appreciation that they are automatic and not in our conscious control, and that they are very quick (Van der Kolk, 2006). By the time a signal of danger arrives in the neocortex, the amygdala has already received the signal and initiated activation of the ANS and our body is being flooded with cortisol and adrenalin, increasing our heart rate, making our breathing shallow, narrowing our visual field, and affecting our gut and liver in preparation for fight or flight. Our processes of thinking are far too slow when danger is present.

The Riverbank Metaphor

In the therapeutic context, Michael White proposed an image of a person's experience of trauma as one of them being swept along in the turmoil of a fast-flowing river, not knowing what is up and what is down. When the person is being tumbled around in the river, it is not the time for meaning making. We need to secure their place on the riverbank and from this solid ground there can then be the opportunity to look upstream and downstream, and to reflect and begin to make sense of what is going on (White, 2006).

I began by asking Alice about the things that she normally did that helped to keep her calm and we were shortly into a discussion of the only pastime she had where she felt she could relax, and that was tending to her small but hardy garden on the balcony of her apartment. I was keen to stay with the account of her interest in gardening, not only with the intention of 'making her comfortable' but more because I wanted to establish a different story of Alice that was free of the influence of the history of abuse and the distress. I enquired into what it took to establish a garden in the somewhat hostile environment of a balcony; how she felt when she was in her garden; how long she had had the interest in gardening. She spoke of practices of dedication, of tending and caring for, especially in the harsh summers, and also of believing that a dead-looking cutting would one day be a bush that was full of flowers. This last comment became a statement from Alice that "*you have to believe that things can grow and change even in the most unlikely circumstances.*" I enquired into the history of both the practical skills of being able to keep things alive and also into the history of this skill of knowing that *things can change and grow even in the most unlikely circumstances.* This seemed to me to be a possible significant life skill that Alice had developed and it turned out to be something that we came back to time and again in the course of our therapeutic conversations.

Alice went on to speak of connections with an elderly neighbor throughout her childhood and of how she often took refuge there when things were really bad at home. Alice remembered a time when she was about 11 coming across Mrs. Beresford kneeling on the path and gently running her hands over the clumps of tiny daisy that were flowering in the crevasses of the cement path and in every available spot in the yard. Mrs. B called Alice over and got her to kneel down and run her hand over the tiny but hardy flowers. "*See how something so beautiful and delicate can grow in the cracks of cement,*" she said. "*It doesn't seem possible but it is!*"

Alice was calmer now and there was a difference in her tone and her face. Having an appreciation of the impact of negative affect (cortisol, adrenaline) on a person's ability to engage in meaning making and to be able to make new connections in the frontal cortex has supported me to spend more time in developing these stories of self that are different to what is problematic (Beaudoin & Zimmerman, 2011). Knowing also that the release of neurochemicals such as serotonin and dopamine that are evinced in positive affect provide an optimal context for new learning has contributed to my practice of taking more time in this before embarking on exploration of the concerns. I began to talk with Alice about her coming to meet with me and how that was for her, and what we might agree to do if things got shaky at any point. We resolved to have the talking about the garden as a place that we could go when or if Alice felt the agitation starting to rise.

Fight or Flight; Freeze or Appease

The theory of a 'fight or flight' that came to be described through the action of the ANS was first described by American physiologist Walter B Canon in the 1920s (Canon, 1932). For many decades the 'fight or flight' response has been well known in the public discourse and even now is often considered the *only* response we make to threat. Since the 1980s however, other equally protective responses have been determined and described as ways of ensuring survival. These are the freeze or appease responses. We have an acutely tuned system of evaluating the degree of threat and, if it is determined that we are not able to either fight or flee from a threatening other that is larger and more powerful than us, then the automatic response of immobility or freezing is the one most likely to aid our survival. Or we will try to appease the threat by giving the attacker something they want and making it clear that we are not a threat (Marks, 1987).

When 'fight or flight' is put forward as *the* response, there can be an internalized belief amongst people who 'froze' or 'appeased' that, because they did not fight or manage to get away when subjected to attack, they were somehow not 'normal.' This has contributed to many women and adult survivors of childhood sexual abuse taking on a belief that they were weak or bad because they did not manage to prevent the attack. Having this in mind has led me to share some of this knowledge with women who have experienced the trauma of abuse. All of the responses of the ANS are non-conscious and automatic reactions that take place in all functioning humans when faced with an overwhelming threat, and the primary purpose of all of them is to enable us to survive the situation. It is the meaning that is made of these responses when the threat has passed that is of concern to us as therapists.

The Role of Language in Memory

When we consider a memory that we have of a past non-stressful event such as a childhood birthday party or an outing to a favorite place, we are generally able to describe what happened and to reflect on the significance of that event; we may be able to re-evoke some of the emotions that are woven into that experience of the past and to describe them. These memories are based on language, though with a complex interplay of non-verbal or felt memories, and being verbal, they are stored in the explicit memory system.

According to Van der Kolk et al., as a consequence of high levels of stress under threat, our verbally based memory system can go 'off-line' (Van der Kolk, 1998). As fear increases, levels of cortisol have an impact on the language centers of the brain. It is much more useful for us to give hyper-vigilant attention to the sensory cues in the environment: the visual, olfactory, auditory, kinesthetic non-verbal experience. This includes the physical sensations in our body and the strong emotions that are telling us that we are in danger and that help us to make rapid assessment of the level of threat. Once the threat has passed however, we are left with these implicit memories of the fear experience and, because they are not anchored in language, there is a risk that any aspect of a current situation that reminds us of the trauma can trigger these traumatic memories.

Implicit memories are non-conscious in that they cannot be consciously recalled and so the emotional response to a threatening situation is not available to be recalled or verbalized. 'Explicit' memories by contrast are conscious memories that have words to them and that are accessible to being recalled intentionally through engagement of the cortical systems of the brain. They are also contextual in that they involve the recalling of multiple aspects of an event or situation, such as where, when and what happened and who else was involved. As a consequence of trauma, memories can be fragmented or lost or not stored in the most useful place. Some aspects of trauma remain encoded in the form of emotional pain, and from here they are able to invade everyday situations where they set off powerful responses that are often inappropriate to the actual situation. The pain is re-experienced and it doesn't make sense.

Experiences of pain can be rendered meaningful and no longer free to attach themselves to non-threatening circumstances by being brought into the consciousness of the cortical functioning; they can be brought in to the explicit memory system through being languaged. A narrative approach suggests that these felt experiences of pain benefit from being storied, and offers a pathway to stories that are enabling of different responses for the person. This pathway is known as 'absent but implicit' (Carey & Walther, 2009; White, 2000, 2004):

> *There's something wrong with me. I can't seem to stop crying once I start. There's this pain in my chest and it makes it hard to talk. I get overwhelmed at times with this feeling of panic and dread and have awful nightmares. My friend Jenny says I should forget about what happened when I was a kid and get on with my life. I want to get over it, I really do, but it's hopeless. I don't know what to do. I'm so messed up.*

The emotional pain that Alice is experiencing is seen by her as an expression of damage or weakness. Another way of looking at the experience of the pain however is to see it as a 'normal' consequence of the way in which Alice's brain and body have been set up to respond to threat and danger. Our brains are organized to be tremendously efficient at learning what is dangerous and so these experiences of threat are encoded very quickly and lastingly as 'emotional' memories in our implicit memory system. While this has been an efficient system for maintaining our survival, it has not proved useful in dealing with the everyday triggers to situations where our wellbeing and safety have been threatened.

The Pathway of the 'Absent but Implicit'

In holding to the double-storied approach to working with people who have experienced traumatic stress, we are interested to understand what the emotional pain that they are experiencing implies. For Alice to express her pain and upset over the abuse that was perpetrated upon her as a child, there must be other meanings of life that she gives great value to that have been violated, otherwise there would not be any tears. We can enter this other story and then develop it in detail as another account of who she is through questions such as: 'What are these tears saying about what is precious and important to you in life that has been violated by what was done? What does the pain tell us about the things that you stand for in life that have been transgressed by what happened to you?'

We can also see that the ongoing pain that Alice is expressing is actually a *response to* what was done and as such it can be conceived of as an action that she is taking (Carey & Walther, 2009). It is some form of position that she is taking on what was done to her: a protest or a resistance or a challenging or questioning of what went on. We can ask questions along the lines of: 'What are the tears and the pain a *response* to? What are you refusing to go along with? What do you think was going on in this situation that was not okay with you?' In posing these questions in this way, we are seeing the pain not as an *effect* of the trauma that Alice has been subjected to, but rather as a *response to* what went on (Yuen, 2007). Seeing the tears as an '*effect of*' contributes to the construction of being helpless and failing to prevent or to get away from the perpetrator. Coming to see that the pain and tears are an active '*response to*' what was going on not only makes sense of the pain but also provides an opening to the development of a different story in which there is the experience of holding strongly to significant and precious understandings of life and of having taken action in accord with these understandings and principles. Focusing on the 'effects of' trauma can imply passivity, while being asked to reflect on ways in which you 'responded to' the trauma feels more active.

Alice replied to my enquiry about what she was responding to with: "*It was terrifying to be left alone in the house with him (her step-dad) when Mum went out to work for her night shifts. I still can't be in a house alone at night. I go into panic mode."* and *"It was like she knew and she abandoned me anyway."* Questions were then asked to elicit a *naming* of her response to these things as an action: What sort of action are the tears and the pain to being made to feel terrified and to being abandoned? How would you say you are responding to these things that were done by your step-dad and your mum?

Naming, Affect Labelling and Lateral Integration

The movement from implicit to explicit memory can be seen as part of a 'vertical integration' between the 'gut reaction' of the limbic system and the cognitive meaning-making processes of the cortical areas of the brain; there is an incorporation of awareness of sensations in the body with the processing of information in the cortex. There is also a further broad delineation of the complex processes of memory and this is in regard to *lateral integration.* The different hemispheres of our brains are engaged in different processes. (Gray, Braver, & Raichle, 2002)

The right hemisphere is largely responsible for the perception of emotion and the processing and analyzing of non-verbal aspects of language. The right hemisphere is also significantly involved in registering the state of our body and in ANS regulation. The left hemisphere is largely involved in logical and linguistic processing and contributes to the encoding of several dimensions of factual memories, including considerations of cause and effect and right versus wrong. It is in the working together of the left and right hemispheres that optimal adaptive states are achieved.

Lieberman et al. (2007) report that being able to name emotion contributes to a reduction in the felt intensity of the emotion, with a corresponding reduction in the activity of the amygdala. In order to contribute to sustainable change in relation to developing a different and more positive and accessible story, the practice of the 'absent but implicit' goes further than just naming. In describing what the person stands for that has been violated, the right prefrontal cortex is engaged through the development of a meaningful narrative. Having emotion taken up into a story line has been shown to be even more powerful in reducing the intensity of the negative affect than simply labelling the affect.

But for Alice to be able to name her tears and pain as active responses to the abuse is not immediately possible. She initially still sees the ongoing experience of pain as a measure of weakness and damage. To move this negative affect into language and meaning requires some careful scaffolding (White, 2007) that supports Alice to come to name for herself what the action is that she has taken. In light of this, I asked Alice if she were happy to go along with having been subjected to a regime of terror, or not. Was she okay with being abandoned by her Mum, or not. Alice responded that she was definitely not happy to go along with what had been done. In this line of enquiry, Alice is being invited to make some discernments in meaning: to work out what the action might be through drawing a distinction with what it is not.

'So, if you are not accepting of what was going on, then what are you doing?' I then asked, to which Alice responded that she was not sure, but that she was clear that she was not going along with what they had done. I offered further scaffolding by putting out some possibilities for Alice's consideration. 'Might this be a refusal or a protest or a resistance or a questioning of some kind?' "*It's a protest and a refusal,*" she eventually responded strongly. "*A determined refusal!*"

For Alice to be able to identify her bodily experiences of fear and anxiety as an active stand against what was done to her bridges from the non-verbal right hemisphere to having this experience languaged in the left hemisphere. There has been both a lateral and vertical integration of the memory, and the story of having taken action in the name of 'protest and refusal' is now available to her to be consciously recalled as an alternative to the single story of the trauma.

But in order for this to be maintained as a different account of herself, we need to contribute to a thickening (White, 2007) of the story that is now getting laid down in memory, and to an embodiment of this new account. The neurobiology of positive affect and the role of the release of serotonin and dopamine and oxytocin ensures that there are markers made to certain memories that are these preferred stories. Understanding this contributed to the careful asking of particular questions that served to bring forward an appreciation that it takes some skill and know-how to be able to protest something that is not okay. 'How is it possible for you to take this action of protesting something that is not okay? How are you able to continue to refuse to just go along with what was done to you?' After some conversation, Alice came to the conclusion that what helped her keep a sense of protest was that "*I knew in my heart it was wrong when it was happening. And I could tell on their faces that they knew it was wrong.*" The questioning took her to an earlier experience of herself where she had always been able to stand her ground at school and at home too. She had lost this sense of herself when the abuse had started, but revisiting it gradually led to it being reclaimed.

Over the course of many conversations, a different story emerged of Alice wanting to reclaim her life from the ongoing effects of the abuse and this reclaiming was seen as a reflection of important understandings of life that she held. "*I want to get my life back. I don't want this stuff to rule me for the rest of my life. It's not fair what they did. Children should be kept safe. Every kid should be able to grow up and be protected,*" she said. "*Everyone has the right grow.*" The developing account was strengthened and thickened through reflection on some of the alternative experiences in her history in which she had taken action that was in line with the themes of protesting and resisting abuse.

Conversations that Alice had had as a 12-year-old with a younger cousin whom she suspected was also being abused, and encouraging her to speak to her school counsellor, were explored in detail. Ideas that had earlier been dismissed of working with children who had had a hard time in life were revived and given new life. The relational histories of these themes were also brought to light and the contributions of significant people to the understandings that "*Children should be kept safe, and everyone has the right grow*" were drawn into the story line.

I wondered what Mrs. Beresford next door might have made of how Alice had taken action in these different ways for the rights of children to be protected and safe and have the right to grow? Alice stated:

> *She always made me feel protected and that I could trust her. It was the only place for a couple of years where I felt like that. And when I think about her loving that things can change grow in the most unlikely places I want to show her that I can grow this different sense of myself out of all of this crap. I never thought I would say it but I can think of myself now as being like those daisies growing and flowering in the cracks of cement.*

Though this is only an excerpt from a particular thread of our conversations, the experience for Alice of coming to these different meanings of the tears and pain and of moving the pain from an implicit experience to an explicit and retrievable memory greatly reduced the power of the trauma experience to invade her life. It made it possible for Alice to have agency in her life and to begin to direct her life in accord with the preferred account that was developed and it became a story that she was able to choose to live by.

Having some understanding of the neurobiology of trauma has brought my attention more to the felt experience in the body of both negative and positive affect and how significant and necessary it is to ensure that my practice forms a substantial bridge to new experience and the development of new and embodied memories. Emotional pain is a consequence of responding to threat and is part of the function of ensuring survival; learning about this as an ability of our brain/body systems rather than it be a personal failing has been highly beneficial for many of the people with whom I have worked. But it is the appreciation of neuroplasticity and how there is always the possibility of being able to develop new stories that are hopeful and life enhancing that continues to energize my work and the lives of those I meet in therapy.

References

Beaudoin, M.-N., & Zimmerman, J. (2011). Narrative therapy and interpersonal neurobiology: Revisiting classic practices, developing new emphases. *Journal of Systemic Therapies, 30*(1), 2–3.

Broks, P. (2004). *Into the silent land: Travels in neuropsychology.* New York, NY: Atlantic Monthly Press.

Canon, W. B. (1932). *The wisdom of the body.* New York, NY: W. W. Norton & Company Inc.

Carey, M., & Walther, S. (2009). The absent but implicit: A map to support therapeutic enquiry. *Family Process, 48*(3), 321–323.

Gray, J., Braver, T., & Raichle, M. (2002). Integration of emotion and cognition in the lateral prefrontal cortex. *PNAS, 99*(6), 4115–4116.

LeDoux, J. (1996). *The emotional brain: The mysterious underpinnings of emotional life.* New York, NY: Simon and Shuster.

Lieberman, D., Eisenberger, N., Crockett, M., Tom, S., Pfeifer, J., & Way, B. (2007, May). Putting feelings into words: Affect labelling disrupts amygdala activity in response to affective stimuli. *Psychological Science, 18*(5), 421–423.

Marks, I. (1987). *Fears, phobias and rituals: Panic, anxiety and their disorders.* New York, NY: Oxford University Press.

Russell, S., & Carey, M. (2004). *Narrative therapy: Responding to your questions.* Adelaide, South Australia: Dulwich Centre Publications.

Van der Kolk, B. (1998). Trauma and memory. In *Psychiatry and Clinical Neurosciences* (pp. S52–S64). New York, NY: Guilford Press.

Van der Kolk, B. (2006). Foreword. In P. Ogden et al. (Eds.), *Trauma and the body: A sensorimotor approach to psychotherapy* (pp. 235–245). New York, NY: W. W. Norton & Company Inc.

White, M. (2000). Re-engaging with history: The absent but implicit. In M. White (Ed.), *Reflections on narrative practice* (pp. 35–58). Adelaide, South Australia: Dulwich Centre Publications.

White, M. (2004). Working with people who are suffering the consequences of multiple trauma: A narrative perspective. *International Journal of Narrative Therapy and Community Work,* (2004 No. 1), 47–48. Adelaide, South Australia: Dulwich Centre Publications.

White, M. (2006). Responding to children who have experienced significant trauma: A narrative perspective. In M. White & A. Morgan (Eds.), *Narrative therapy with children and their families* (pp. 87–92). Adelaide, South Australia: Dulwich Centre Publications.

White, M. (2007). *Maps of narrative practice.* New York, NY: W. W. Norton & Company Inc.

Yuen, A. (2007). Discovering children's responses to trauma: A response-based narrative practice. *The International Journal of Narrative Therapy and Community Work, 4,* 3–18.

4 Supporting Young Children Visited by Big Emotions

Mindfulness, Emotion Regulation, and Neurobiology

Sara Marlowe

Neuroscience research shows that mindfulness practice can mediate our experience of strong emotions and lead to changes in the brain that nurture emotion regulation and overall wellbeing. This chapter will present mindfulness-based practices, grounded in neurobiology, for clinicians, educators and parents to support children with emotion regulation. Through the stories of three children, mindfulness activities that develop somatic awareness of emotions, reduce reactivity to big emotions when they come to visit and cultivate positive emotions will be shared.

Brooke, 6 years old, loves to sing, dance, swim and play. Sometimes however, Mr. Frustration comes to visit, especially when she has difficulty completing a task. He shows up in her throat and eventually takes her fun away. Nine-year-old Tyron loves to skate, cuddle with his cat, play with his friends and draw. The Angry Ninjas come around mostly at school when he feels left out by his friends. Chao-xing, 7 years old, loves to play piano, build Lego, read and ride her bike, but when the Worrier-Worrys show up, they keep her head spinning so fast she can't seem to do anything . . . not even sleep!

Just like adults, children can at times get overwhelmed by strong emotions and react in ways that unintentionally lead to more difficulties in their lives. Mindfulness practice is an effective way to support adults and children to 'ride the waves' of big emotions when they come to visit. When we learn to hold our attention on present-moment experiences, we become intentional participants in not only choosing how we respond to the world around us, but also in changing our brain (Fisher & Ogden, 2011).

Since learning about neurobiology, I include the following elements in my individual, family and group work with children: development of somatic awareness of emotions; the practice of naming emotional experiences; mindfulness as a way to calm reactivity to big emotions when they come to visit; and the cultivation of positive emotions as a practice to access and further develop the brain's positive neural pathways. This chapter will share some of the playful practices developed to support Brooke, Tyron, Chao-xing—and other children—with emotion regulation when visited by big emotions.

Mindfulness Practice, Emotion Regulation, and the Brain

Advances in neurobiology demonstrate that an act of the mind is capable of rewiring the brain (Schwartz & Begley, 2003). Mindfulness, which is an act of the mind, leads to neuroplastic changes in the structure and function of brain regions involved in the regulation of attention, self-awareness and emotion (Tang, Holzel, & Posner, 2015). It has the potential to increase subjective wellbeing, improve behavioral regulation, reduce emotional reactivity (Keng, Smoski, & Robins, 2011) and enhance self-regulation (Hölzel et al., 2011). It also has a positive impact on the neural expression of emotion regulation in the brain.

Bishop et al. (2004) define mindfulness as paying attention to one's present-moment experience and relating to it with a curious, open and accepting stance. Bringing this quality of attention to one's internal experiences in the present moment helps us to notice when we are getting 'hooked' by difficult emotions, unhelpful thought patterns or discomfort in the body. The act of observing our experiences creates space to more purposefully respond to challenges—in ways we prefer—rather than reacting automatically. Learning to face emotional situations with a focus on present-moment experience has an overall emotional regulating effect by reducing activity in brain regions involved in emotion processing when faced with negative stimuli (Lutz et al., 2014). Williams (2010) found that eight weeks of mindfulness practice is sufficient to alter the ways in which emotions are regulated and processed in the brain.

The experience of intense emotions can send us into survival mode—'Flight, Fight, or Freeze'—where blood flow to the prefrontal cortex (PFC) is reduced and we are unable to engage in logical discussion or problem-solving. Bringing mindful awareness to body sensations and emotions can be helpful in such situations to calm the amygdala and reengage the PFC (Kozlowska, Walker, McLean, & Carrive, 2015). Mindfulness increases our recovery from emotional challenges, increases our tolerance to negative affect and teaches us to observe emotions as "innocuous sensory information" rather than as threats requiring an immediate response (Farb et al., 2010, p. 31). It is associated with decreased activations in regions related to emotional arousal (Lutz et al., 2014) and sometimes shrinkage of the amygdala itself, the brain's alarm signal (Taren, Creswell, & Gianardos, 2013). Mindfulness is also linked to increased activation in the dorsolateral and dorsomedial prefrontal cortex, which are regulatory structures in the brain (Tang et al., 2015). The aforementioned research has been with adults; however, when adapted to be age-appropriate, mindfulness has the potential to grow neural circuitry that will support emotional regulation across the lifespan (Zelazo & Lyons, 2012).

Mindfulness and Body Awareness

Simply the act of exhaling engages the parasympathetic nervous system, unconsciously signaling the body to relax (Hanson, 2009). Teaching children fun ways to engage in deep breathing can be relaxing; for example, blowing bubbles, pinwheels and cotton balls, or playing with Hoberman Spheres.[1] Mindfulness, however, is more than deep breathing and relaxation. It also encourages body awareness by increasing activity in the insula and structural properties of brain regions connected to body awareness (Farb et al., 2007). Since information from the body informs us of how we are feeling (Baldini, Parker, Nelson, & Siegel, 2014), cultivating body awareness supports the development of emotion regulation (Carré, Guillaume, Duclos, Bayot, & Shankland, 2015). Overall, mindfulness strengthens the observing part of the brain so we can notice and respond to our bodily reactions rather than having them take over (Ogden, 2013). When children practice noticing body sensations, they also lay a foundation for developing awareness of more complex aspects of their subjective experience, namely thoughts and emotions (Zelazo & Lyons, 2012).

Mindfulness Practice with Children

Research over the past decade has found mindfulness practice to benefit children (Shonin, Van Gordon, & Griffiths, 2012) and it has expanded into educational and mental health settings (Flook et al., 2010; Jennings, Frank, Snowberg, Coccia, & Greenberg, 2013; Schonert-Reichl et al., 2015). Mindfulness with children can improve behavioral regulation (Flook et al., 2010), foster academic learning (Weare, 2013), reduce anxiety (Semple, Reid, & Miller, 2005), increase executive function (Diamond & Lee, 2011), reduce stress (Rempel, 2012) and promote overall resilience (Lantierri, 2008). Whether it is for supporting children with school-related issues, mental health challenges and anxiety, or for general wellbeing, many parents are now looking to mindfulness for their children. The remainder of this chapter will present mindfulness activities developed for children that aim to integrate the neurobiology of emotion regulation.

Noticing and Naming Big Emotions: The Inside Flashlight

A flashlight is a playful metaphor for focusing attention. In this practice, children are invited to shine their flashlight on their inner experiences—to spend some time looking *inside* and bring a curiosity to what they observe in terms of body sensations, thoughts and emotions. It supports them to practice body awareness and notice and name emotions, which calms the amygdala and reduces reactivity (Lieberman et al., 2007). Further, engaging the left hemisphere of the brain to *name* our emotional experiences in the right hemisphere helps to *tame* them (Siegel & Payne Bryson, 2011). Sharing information with children about how the brain works increases their interest in engaging in mindfulness practices and decreases their feelings of self-blame when strong feelings visit.

The following passage is from *The Inside Flashlight*, a story I wrote to introduce this practice:

> *When trouble takes you for a ride, close your eyes and look inside.*
> *What thoughts are there? What feelings too? What is your body*
>   *telling you?*
> *Take a breath or two or four, do nothing less, do nothing more.*
> *Then take another look inside, and give a name to what you find.*

To begin, children are asked what flashlights are used for—common answers include to "help us see in the dark," or "help you find your way." A real flashlight is then directed on a particular spot in the room and people are asked to notice 10 or 12 things where the flashlight is shining. Children are often amazed at how many different things they see when focusing their attention in this way. Next, participants lie down on a yoga mat or sit on a chair or cushion, and are asked to imagine shining a flashlight *inside* and bring that same focused attention to their internal experiences. Below is a loose script for the practice that can be adapted according to the ages and level of focus of the children. Aspects of this practice (such as awareness of breath, body awareness, thoughts and emotions) can be taught over multiple sessions to scaffold the development of mindfulness skills. It follows well after children have had some practice observing their breath.

- We begin with bringing our attention to our breath, taking a few soft and deep breaths. Then, gently following our inbreath and our outbreath.
- Next, imagine switching on your flashlight and looking around *inside*. Bringing your attention to your breath, as if shining a flashlight where you notice your breath. Observing the movement of the breath. Quietly saying to yourself "in, out," as you breath in and out.
- Next, bringing your attention to sensations you notice in your body.

  - What do your fingers and hands feel like? Are they tight? Loose? Warm? Cool? How about your toes? Legs? Your back? Your shoulders? What might you notice about the body when you shine your flashlight of attention there?
  - Do you notice any sensations in your belly? Is it gurgly? Tight? Hungry?
  - How about your heartbeat? Is it fast and jumpy? Or slow and steady?

- What thoughts do you notice? Are they fast? Quiet? Just watching them come and go.
- What feelings do you notice? What might you call them? Sleepiness? Comfort? Restlessness? Boredom? Curiosity? Worry? Frustration? Do you feel them somewhere in the body? Perhaps there is one that catches your attention the most. What might you call it? You could even say quietly to yourself, "Worry is visiting" for example (or whichever emotion you have named), and then just letting it be there.
- Then, shining the *inside* flashlight back on your breath. Following your breath for a few more moments as you breathe in and breathe out.
- You can use your flashlight to practice observing and naming what's going on inside throughout the day, during challenging times and during fun times as well. By naming our emotions, we can tame their potential effect on us.

Making Inside Flashlights: Integrating art is an engaging way to teach mindfulness to children (Coholic, 2011) and a tangible reminder to practice. Children can make a flashlight keychain using shrink film[2] to carry with them as a reminder to observe and name their internal experiences (see Figure 4.1). Or they can color and laminate a paper outline of a flashlight with the passage from the story above printed on the back. Parents can use this metaphor to support their children to observe and name their internal experiences.

Tyron used his inside flashlight primarily at school, where the Angry Ninjas showed up the most. He talked with his parents about how tightness in his belly became a clue that the Angry Ninjas were close by. After some time, Tyron often recognized when the Angry Ninjas were about to, or had just, shown up. Taking some deep breaths, talking to a teacher or reading a loving note from his mother were ways he found helpful to

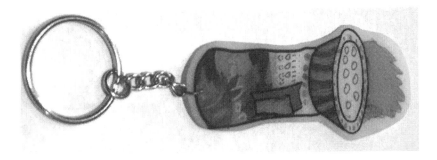

Figure 4.1 Inside flashlight keychain made by a 7 year old

keep them from overwhelming him. The inside flashlight practice supported Tyron to slow down the Angry Ninjas' automatic attack and to make more purposeful choices in responding to the experience of anger and hurt that often came when he felt excluded by his friends. By learning to bring awareness to the emotional and physical experience of the Angry Ninjas, Tyron was training his brain to be able to observe them, rather than automatically reacting to get rid of the feeling. After Tyron named his problem with explosive anger "The Angry Ninjas," he was less reactive and more able to access his PFC to implement useful strategies when they showed up.

Naming the anger separated Tyron from the problem and enabled him to speak more freely about it (White & Epston, 1990) and to create space to explore his preferences, hopes, values, skills and alternatives to the problem story (Duvall & Béres, 2011), as illustrated in the following dialogue:

Mom (M):   His teacher said he didn't explode and get into a fight with his friends like last time.

Tyron (T):   Yeah, the Angry Ninjas didn't show up much at school this week. They usually show up all the time.

Sara (S):   So, this week the Angry Ninjas showed up less at school?

T: Yeah, only once or twice. Instead of every second!

S: Wow, that's a lot less than last week. What kept them away so much?

T: When they came last week, I talked about it with my mom on the way home.

M: We talked about how he might use the inside flashlight to notice when the Angry Ninjas are about to show up. He talked *a lot* more than when we used to talk about "why he was so angry." Once we got home, we reviewed our list about how to win a battle with the Angry Ninjas. And every day now, I put a note saying, "I love you," in his bag or pocket.

T: Yeah, I read mom's note and tried a couple things as soon as I felt them making my belly tight.

S: A couple of things?

T: When my belly got tight, I read the note from my mom and took a few breaths. I told myself "the Angry Ninjas are coming." I then told my teacher, who has agreed to help me out.

S: Was this a more useful way to respond to the Angry Ninjas?

T: Yes.

S: How come?

T: They didn't take over. I didn't get in trouble and kept playing with my friends.

S: Ah yes. You have talked a lot about how important playing with your friends is to you.

Conversations then continued with Tyron and his family that explored his preferences for getting along well with friends, his values around friend-ship, his skills in making and keeping friends, and the possibilities that this new way of relating to the Angry Ninjas were opening up for him.

The inside flashlight practice also supported Brooke in developing somatic awareness of her emotional experiences, particularly frustration. She learned to recognize that a hot face and a thumpy-bumpy heartbeat were signs that Mr. Frustration was about to show up. The process of naming Mr. Frustration and telling the story of his impact loosened his grip. She was then more able to draw from her list of calming strategies that she developed with her parents for when he bothered her.

Calming Big Emotions When They Come to Visit: Stillness Snow Globes

We all have times when strong emotions take over and we act in ways that are not our preference. With mindfulness practice, we can learn to notice our early warning signs for when we may be about to become overwhelmed by strong emotions and draw on ways to calm ourselves. Snow globes, a traditional metaphor in mindfulness practice, can be a playful calming activity for children. They can illustrate how when we are able to settle our thoughts, emotions and body sensations, even though they don't disappear, we can see more clearly (Willard, 2010). When strong emotions do take over, using a snow globe can support children to calm their mind and body and help them to reconnect with something they hold dear. Children can make their own snow globes and include in them images or words of things in their life that are important to them.

Making Stillness Snow Globes: Children are given a 'photo snow globe' into which photos are inserted, some colored paper and markers. First, they cut two pieces of colored paper using the template inside the globe. Next, they bring to mind something that is positive for them—a supportive person, a pet, an activity they like to do or kind words they or someone else may say to them, for example. They draw or write these positive things onto the pieces of paper and insert them vertically into the snow globe. Some examples of words from children in my work include, 'breathe, calm, and love,' and images have included 'playing soccer, family, hugging a parent and snuggling a pet.'

Next, children are invited to shake their snow globes and quietly observe the snowflakes as they settle to the bottom. When they are swirling, the images inside are obscured, and can only be seen clearly once the flakes have settled. Children often comment on how watching the snowflakes set-tle helps them to feel more settled. They can also play with matching their body movement with the snowflakes, as they swirl around when shaken, and then slowly settle to the floor. This latter activity supports children to embody the feeling of unsettledness, followed by settling into stillness.

Children can shake their snow globe when they notice big emotions coming to visit. They can even imagine that these snowflakes represent the challenging thoughts/feelings or body sensations that are visiting them. They can watch them settle and notice their pleasant image or words become more visible. They can think about where, and when, they might use their snow globe and consider a place to keep it handy. Sometimes parents even 'borrow' their child's snow globe and shake it up before responding to their child when they are feeling an intense emotion. It helps them to calm potential reactivity and be more intentional in responding to their child.

Chao-xing found her stillness snow globe to be particularly helpful when she was experiencing 'The Worrier-Worrys' that showed up at school and often before bed. She drew her pet gecko and the word 'love' inside of her snow globe. She kept her snow globe by her bed and would shake it as part of her going-to-bed routine, which helped to calm the Worrier-Worrys so that she could more easily fall asleep. Chao-xing also took her snow globe to school on days where she anticipated the Worrier-Worrys might show up—particularly when she had a spelling quiz. Shaking her snow globe and watching the snowflakes settle helped to settle her swirling and jittery thoughts so that she could focus more on her spelling.

Cultivating Positive Emotions: Noticing Positive Experiences and Practicing Self-Kindness

It is well documented that the human brain has a negativity bias, which can lead us to focus more on problems at the expense of noticing what is going well. In general, it takes at least a three-to-one ratio of positivity to negativity to keep the brain in balance, given that negative emotional states resonate with greater force and energy (Fredrickson, 2009). Cultivating positive emotions, however, can help us to better cope with the negative ones (Tugade & Fredrickson, 2007). It strengthens regions and connections in the brain that lead to an increased sense of optimism and possibility (Davidson, 2012) and develops the positive neural networks in the brain (Hanson, 2013; Harnett & Dawe, 2012). We can do this by noticing positive experiences, practicing compassion and kindness, and expressing gratitude for things great or small (Benn, Akiva, Robert, & Roeser, 2012; Osimo, 2009).

Bringing Awareness to Positive Experiences: Children and families can practice observing pleasant moments throughout the day, share them with each other and express gratitude for having experienced them. During a pleasant moment, people can bring attention to thoughts, emotions and body sensations. Bringing awareness to the 'felt-sense' details supports pleasant experiences to be more vivid and thus more solidified into memory (Hanson, 2009). As a way to deepen the positive experience, people can recall these pleasant events at a later time—ostensibly reliving them in their mind and body (Hanson, 2013). Charades offers a playful way for groups and families to practice embodying pleasant events. In a group setting, families can mime a pleasant experience they shared and have other members try to guess the experience. In this way, they are physically embodying the pleasant experience. Parents often report feeling more hopeful and viewing their child in a more positive light when they practice noticing pleasant experiences. They recognize the problem is only a part of their life and they are doing well in spite of its existence.

Each day, Tyron and his mother would talk about a positive moment before discussing any challenges that may have occurred. She might ask him about the funniest, silliest or most proud part of his day. She said this practice led to less tension on the drive home and more connection between the two of them.

Practicing Self-kindness and Compassion: Practicing compassion and kindness is another way to cultivate positive emotions and help loosen the grip of problems in our lives. Problems can lead us to feel badly about ourselves and practicing self-compassion provides a way to counter the negative self-image that often accompanies problems and labels. Self-kindness and compassion practice buffers us against the impact of negative events (Leary, Tate, Adams, Allen, & Hancock, 2007) and generates positive emotions by embracing negative ones (Germer & Neff, 2013).

One fun way for families to practice this with young children is through the song, 'May We be Happy,'[3] which draws on traditional loving, kindness and compassion practice drawing on the repetition of phrases wishing ourselves and others to be happy and free from suffering. The story, 'My New Best Friend,' written by myself, also teaches children how to be kind and compassionate towards themselves.

Brooke's family reported that once she started a daily practice of printing a kind message to herself in a kindness journal, Mr. Frustration started to step back. Brooke was able to draw on these kind messages during difficult tasks to remind herself she was doing her best.

Summary

This chapter presented mindfulness-based practices to nurture children's emotional regulation by developing somatic awareness of emotions, encouraging the naming of emotional experiences and cultivating positive emotions. These activities are ideally shared with an attitude of *planting seeds* of mindfulness (Hanh, 2011); letting go of specific expectations of how children *should* respond and instead being flexible to adapt them based on children's responses in the present moment. Starting to practice mindfulness in childhood can not only support children in the moment, but also develop neural circuitry that will support them throughout their lives when big emotions come to visit.

Notes

1. Hoberman Spheres are geometric-shaped toys that children can expand and contract while matching their breath with the movement of the sphere.
2. Shrink film is plastic art material that shrinks to half its size and hardens once it is baked.
3. The lyrics and melody to 'May We be Happy' can be found at www.mindful families.ca.

References

Baldini, L. L., Parker, S. C., Nelson, B. W., & Siegel, D. J. (2014). The clinician as neuroarchitect: The importance of mindfulness and presence in clinical practice. *Clinical Social Work Journal, 42*, 218–227.

Benn, R., Akiva, T., Robert, S. A., & Roeser, W. (2012). Mindfulness training effects for parents and educators of children with special needs. *Developmental Psychology, 48*(5), 1476–1487.

Bishop, S. R., Lau, M., Shapiro, S., Carlson, L., Anderson, N. D., Carmody, J., . . . & Devins, G. (2004). Mindfulness: A proposed operational definition. *Clinical Psychology: Science and Practice, 11*(3), 230–241.

Carré, A., Guillaume, P., Duclos, J., Bayot, M., & Shankland, R. (2015). From body to emotion regulation: A psychometric study. Conference Paper. Retrieved from http://www.researchgate.net/publication/277726654_From_Body_to_Emotion_Regulation_A_Psychometric_Study

Coholic, D. (2011). Exploring the feasibility and benefits of arts-based mindfulness-awareness and resilience. *Child & Youth Care Forum, 40*, 303–317.

Davidson, R. J. (2012). *The emotional life of your brain: How its unique patterns affect the way you think, feel, and live—and how you can change them*. New York, NY: Plume.

Diamond, A., & Lee, K. (2011). Interventions shown to aid executive function development in children 4–12 years old. *Science, 333*(6045), 959–964.

Duvall, J., & Béres, L. (2011). *Innovations in narrative therapy: Connecting practice, training and research*. New York, NY: W. W. Norton & Company Inc.

Farb, N. A. S., Anderson, A. K., Mayberg, H. S., Bean, J., McKeon, D., & Segal, Z. V. (2010). Minding one's emotions: Mindfulness training alters the neural expression of sadness. *Emotion, 10*(1), 25–33.

Farb, N. A. S., Segal, Z. V., Mayberg, H., Bean, J., McKeon, D., Fatima, Z., & Anderson, A. K. (2007). Attending to the present: Mindfulness meditation reveals distinct neural modes of self-reference. *Social Cognitive & Affective Neuroscience, 2*(4), 313–322.

Fisher, J., & Ogden, P. (2011). Case study, breaking free: A mind-body approach to retraining the brain. *Psychotherapy Networker, 35*(2), 57–63.

Flook, L., Smalley, S., Kitil, M. J., Galla, B. M., Kaiser-Greenland, S., Locke, J., . . . & Kasari, C. (2010). Effects of mindful awareness practices on executive functions in elementary school children. *Journal of Applied School Psychology, 26*, 70–95.

Fredrickson, B. (2009). *Positivity: Top-notch research reveals the 3 to 1 ratio that will change your life*. New York, NY: Three Rivers.

Germer, C., & Neff, K. (2013). Self-compassion in clinical practice. *Journal of Clinical Psychology: In Session, 69*(8), 856–867.

Hanh, T. N. (2011). *Planting seeds: Practicing mindfulness with children.* Berkeley, CA: Parallax Press.

Hanson, R. (2009). *Buddha's brain: The practical neuroscience of happiness, love & wisdom.* Oakland, CA: New Harbinger Publications Inc.

Hanson, R. (2013). *Hardwiring happiness: The new brain science of contentment, calm, and confidence.* New York, NY: Harmony Books.

Harnett, P. H., & Dawe, S. (2012). The contribution of mindfulness-based therapies for children and families and proposed conceptual integration. *Child and Adolescent Mental Health, 17*(4), 195–208.

Hölzel, B. K., Lazar, S. W., Gard, T., Schuman-Olivier, Z., Vago, D. R., & Ott, U. (2011). How does mindfulness meditation work? Proposing mechanisms of action from a conceptual and neural perspective. *Perspectives on Psychological Science, 6*(6), 537–559.

Jennings, P. A., Frank, J. L., Snowberg, K. E., Coccia, M. A., & Greenberg, M. T. (2013). Improving classroom learning environments by cultivating awareness and resilience in education (care): Results of a randomized controlled trial. *School Psychology Quarterly, 28*(4), 374–390.

Keng, S., Smoski, M. J., & Robins, C. J. (2011). Effects of mindfulness on psychological health: A review of empirical studies. *Clinical Psychology Review, 31,* 1041–1056.

Kozlowska, K., Walker, P., McLean, L., & Carrive, P. (2015). Fear and the defense cascade: Clinical implications and management. *Harvard Review of Psychiatry, 23*(4), 263–287.

Lantierri, L. (2008). *Building emotional intelligence: Techniques to cultivate inner strength in children.* Colorado: Sounds True.

Leary, M., Tate, E., Adams, C., Allen, A., & Hancock, J. (2007). Self-compassion and reactions to unpleasant self-relevant events: The implications of treating oneself kindly. *Journal of Personality and Social Psychology, 92*(5), 887–904.

Lieberman, M. D., Eisenberger, N. I., Crockett, M. J., Tom, S. M., Pfeifer, J. H., & Way, B. M. (2007). Putting feelings into words: Affect labeling disrupts amygdala activity in response to affective stimuli. *Association for Psychological Science, 18*(5), 421–428.

Lutz, J., Herwig, U., Opialla, S., Hittmeyer, A., Jancke, L., Rufer, M., . . . & Bruhl, A. B. (2014). Mindfulness and emotion regulation: An fMRI study. *Social Cognitive & Affective Neuroscience, 9*(6), 776–785.

Ogden, P. (2013). *How neurobiology changed the way we view the treatment of trauma.* Retrieved from https://www.google.ca/#q=Ogden%2C+P.+(2013).+How+neurobiology+changed+the+way+we+view+the+treatment+of+trauma.+

Osimo, J. (2009). *An examination of neuroscience findings in attention, self-regulation, mindfulness, and narrative language: Potential links in psychotherapeutic interventions.* (Doctoral Dissertation). Pepperdine University. ProQuest Dissertations and Theses.

Rempel, K. D. (2012). Mindfulness for children and youth: A review of the literature with an argument for school-based implementation. *Canadian Journal of Counselling and Psychotherapy, 46*(3), 201–220.

Schonert-Reichl, K. A., Oberle, E., Lawlor, M. S., Abbott, D., Thomson, K., Oberlander, T. F., & Diamond, A. (2015). Enhancing cognitive and social–emotional development through a simple-to-administer mindfulness-based school program for elementary school children: A randomized controlled trial. *Developmental Psychology, 51*(1), 52–66.

Schwartz, J. M., & Begley, S. (2003). *The mind and the brain: Neuroplasticity and the power of mental force.* New York, NY: Harper Collins Publishing.

Semple, R., Reid, E. F. G., & Miller, L. (2005). Treating anxiety with mindfulness. *Journal of Cognitive Psychotherapy: An International Quarterly, 19*(4), 379–392.

Shonin, E., Van Gordon, W., & Griffiths, M. D. (2012). The health benefits of mindfulness-based interventions for children and adolescents. *Education and Health, 30*(4), 95–98.

Siegel, D., & Payne Bryson, T. (2011). *The whole-brain child: 12 revolutionary strategies to nurture your child's developing mind.* New York, NY: Random House.

Tang, Y., Holzel, B. K., & Posner, M. I. (2015). The neuroscience of mindfulness meditation. *Nature Reviews Neuroscience, 16*, 213–225.

Taren, A. A., Creswell, D., & Gianardos, P. J. (2013). Dispositional mindfulness co-varies with smaller amygdala and caudate volumes in community adults. *PLoS One, 8*(5), 1–7.

Tugade, M. M., & Fredrickson, B. L. (2007). Regulation of positive emotions: Emotion regulation strategies that promote resilience. *Journal of Happiness Studies, 8*(3), 311–333.

Weare, K. (2013). Developing mindfulness with children and young people: A review of the evidence and policy context. *Journal of Children's Services, 8*(2), 141–153.

White, M., & Epston, D. (1990). *Narrative means to therapeutic ends.* New York, NY: W. W. Norton & Company Inc.

Willard, C. (2010). *Child's mind: Mindfulness practices to help our children be more focused, calm, and relaxed.* Berkeley, CA: Parallax Press.

Williams, J. M. G. (2010). Mindfulness and psychological process. *Emotion, 10*, 1–7.

Zelazo, P. D., & Lyons, K. E. (2012). The potential benefits of mindfulness training in early childhood: A developmental social cognitive neuroscience perspective. *Child Development Perspectives, 6*(2), 154–160.

5   Insights on Positive Change

An Exploration of the Link between Drama Therapy and Neural Networks

Pam Dunne

People gravitate towards the creative arts therapies because they feel a connection to the arts and are curious to explore, test, and discover alternative views in which to look at their problems and learn how to forge new, preferred pathways in their life. As a seasoned creative therapist, I've spent the last 25 years in the innovative field of drama therapy, while simultaneously incorporating the other creative arts in my work and practice. In 1995, I developed narradrama, a specific method in drama therapy that integrates drama, narrative, and the creative arts.

In order to understand how narradrama works, three central drama therapy principles must first be understood: 1) dramatic embodiment, or the physical expression of a role; 2) dramatic projection, which is the externalization of some aspect of the client's internal voice; and 3) distancing, which refers to the client's sense of closeness or detachment from their thoughts and feelings. Dramatic embodiment, dramatic projection, and distancing via a role provides a safe structure in which to help clients express their emotions, but not be overwhelmed by them, so that they may find balance.

Through narradrama, I have been able to offer a unique therapeutic experience to my clients, while also continuing to be a part of the ever-growing field of the creative arts therapies, narrative therapy, and the social sciences that fuel ongoing curiosity, learning, and refinement—not only within my practice, but in my body of work as a therapist.

Five years ago, while attending my first-ever interpersonal neurobiology conference, I had an "aha" moment while sitting amongst the thousand other attendees in a large auditorium at UCLA. Listening to Dr. Dan Siegel, the keynote speaker, I found myself completely absorbed, hanging onto every sentence. The connection between interpersonal neurobiology and narradrama was undeniable. I left the conference that day flooded with energy, excitement, and exhaustion—along with *all* of Siegel's books—eager to delve deeper, investigate this connection, and discover how this field would, in turn, inform my practice, my work, and my growth as a therapist.

As I dived into the work of Siegel and interpersonal neurobiology, I also discovered affective neuroscience, or the study of emotional systems in the brain. After spending some time studying these areas, core questions that tied into my own work and practice arose: *What kind of narradrama techniques might help in the strengthening of synaptic connections? What are the effects of positive emotions as part of a therapeutic session?* Eager to find, and implement, the answers, I was drawn back to Siegel's work in interpersonal neurobiology, specifically his research on the strengthening of neural networks. Siegel indicates that through repetition, emotional arousal, novelty, and the careful focus of attention, neural firing can lead to the strengthening of synaptic connections (2011, p. 40). In this chapter, I explore the connection of each of these four areas as it relates to narradrama while detailing what techniques I use to optimize the affective, neural, cognitive, and behavioral benefits that can be achieved.

Repetition

Originally referred to as Hebb's law, you may be familiar with the saying, "as neurons fire together, they wire together." When we have an experience, our neurons become activated. It is within the context of the neurogenesis[1] process in which Siegel (2011) contends, "under the right conditions, neural firing can lead to the strengthening of synaptic connections" (p. 40). The first of the four areas Siegel refers to is repetition. In the therapeutic setting, one way in which repetition can be explored is through the repetition of experience. As a client repeats experiences that contradict their problem-saturated story and negative identity role, and instead repeatedly present an opportunity to experience a unique-outcome story and preferred role, behavior and self-identity descriptions may be able to shift. As Siegel (2011) writes, "our experiences stimulate neural firing and sculpt our emerging synaptic connections" (p. 41). This is how experience changes the structure of the brain itself. In a therapeutic setting, the therapist then works with the client in order to "repeat experiences which reflect their preferences, skills and knowledge. If infused with positive affect, then these neural connections become reinforced and new links are made through the strengthening of synaptic connections" (Beaudoin & Zimmerman, 2011, p. 6).

Preferred Roles

The use of Preferred Roles is integral in narradrama. By repeatedly taking on a positive, preferred role that is connected to a positive emotion, the client can begin to internalize that role, start acting in healthier ways in their everyday lives, and, as Landy (2008) describes, start acting "in ways similar to the role model" (p. 103).

Preferred Role Monologue

In the narradrama exercise, Preferred Role Monologue, the client creates improvised monologues in roles and settings of their own choosing.

This exercise is typically broken up into two different role explorations: the first part begins with a fictional, mythical, and/or fantasy role of their choosing. This can then be followed by second role in which the client plays a preferred version of herself. Often the therapist will aid in the development of these roles and scene settings by asking open-ended questions intended to further broaden possibilities for client exploration in these roles. This exploration lasts several sessions and provides a repeated opportunity for the client to sustain novel, positive experiences within new landscapes, which in turn can help to create new, preferred behaviors in their own life.

To illustrate, Alexis,[2] a woman in her late twenties, begins therapy as she feels despondent about her life, describing herself as unhappy, a failure, and lacking energy to even leave the house. During one of our first sessions together, she describes wishing she were somebody else entirely, the opposite of herself, an "adventurer," she says. After asking several questions that allowed her to further construct who this adventurer was, I invite her to take on this character, who she names Alice the Adventurer, in a preferred role monologue. Throughout our sessions together, Alexis repeatedly explored several monologues while in this role, such as illustrated below, where Alice the Adventurer speaks from high in the sky in a hot-air balloon:

> *"I LOVE it up here. I see a million other places I could go whenever I wish . . . I will watch the ripples in the water from that bridge over there, I will climb that big grassy mountain up there, I will touch clouds and sing with birds and dance with the wind all day long, and then wander as the sun sets and the big moon takes its turn to shine high in the sky."*

At one point in our sessions, Alexis shifts from the role of Alice the Adventurer to playing a realistic role, one that is based on a preferred version of herself. Having spent so much time working in the fantasy role monologue exercises, it is not surprising that some aspects of Alice the Adventurer are clearly present when Alexis plays herself:

> *"I think I'm getting hung up on my problems instead of fixing them. Talking isn't going to change anything. I've got to take action . . . if I want to live the life I want, then I have to grow up and go for it. I want to follow my passions. I want to travel. I want to leave my dead-end job. I want to move forward, towards something better, towards my goals, and into a life I want for myself."*

The marked shift that Alexis makes through her repeated explorations using Preferred Role Monologues aides in her ultimately shifting her own self-identity description. As Cozolino (2016) writes, "humans are capable of imagining alternative selves, creating new narratives to become these selves, and then using narratives as blueprints for changing their lives" (p. 26). Alexis presented as a young woman who self-described as lacking the energy to even leave her own home to an energetic force embracing life and embarking on her next chapter.

Emotional Arousal

The second condition that can aid in the creation of synaptic linkages is emotional arousal, which involves the activation of thoughts and feelings that are associated with physiological or behavioral consequences. Siegel (2011) asserts that when we're not engaged emotionally, the experience is less "memorable," and the structure of the brain is less likely to change (p. 85). Positive emotional arousal results in many benefits (further elaborated on in Chapter 2), as it "opens up our hearts and minds . . . allows us to discover and build new skills, new ties, new knowledge, and new ways of being" (Fredrickson, 2009, pp. 21–24). Creating art and reflecting on it can also arouse emotions. "Sensory inputs activated in art making are processed by thalamic-amygdala visual cortex connections, which contributes to implicit emotional arousal, as well as to explicit emotional awareness and cognitive insight" (Hass-Cohen & Findlay, 2015, p. 191).

Emotional Arousal through Unique Outcomes

Narrative therapy focuses on lived experience through stories and asks questions about the meanings we attach to these stories. Of particular importance is the unique-outcome story, which allows clients to experience being more like the person they prefer. Beaudoin and Zimmerman (2011) emphasize that the more detail and imagery the client reveals about the unique-outcome story, the more significant their emotional involvement (pp. 8–12). One way the researchers found to increase emotional arousal is by asking specific questions about the narrative that involve the client re-experiencing the moment through the details by answering questions such as what they felt in their body at the time and focusing on the thoughts they remembered while experiencing it. In narradrama, clients detail their unique-outcome stories, and thus increase their emotional involvement, through the utilization of dramatic techniques, such as scene setting, interviewing, and enacting. A therapist using narradrama, for example, would first invite the client to create "the where" of the scene with fabrics and/or objects (see Figure 5.1). Then, the client would give the therapist a tour of "the where," verbally detailing the setting. Next, the therapist would initiate a warm-up exercise, such as an interview, with the client in their preferred role. Lastly, the client would begin the actual enactment in their preferred role.

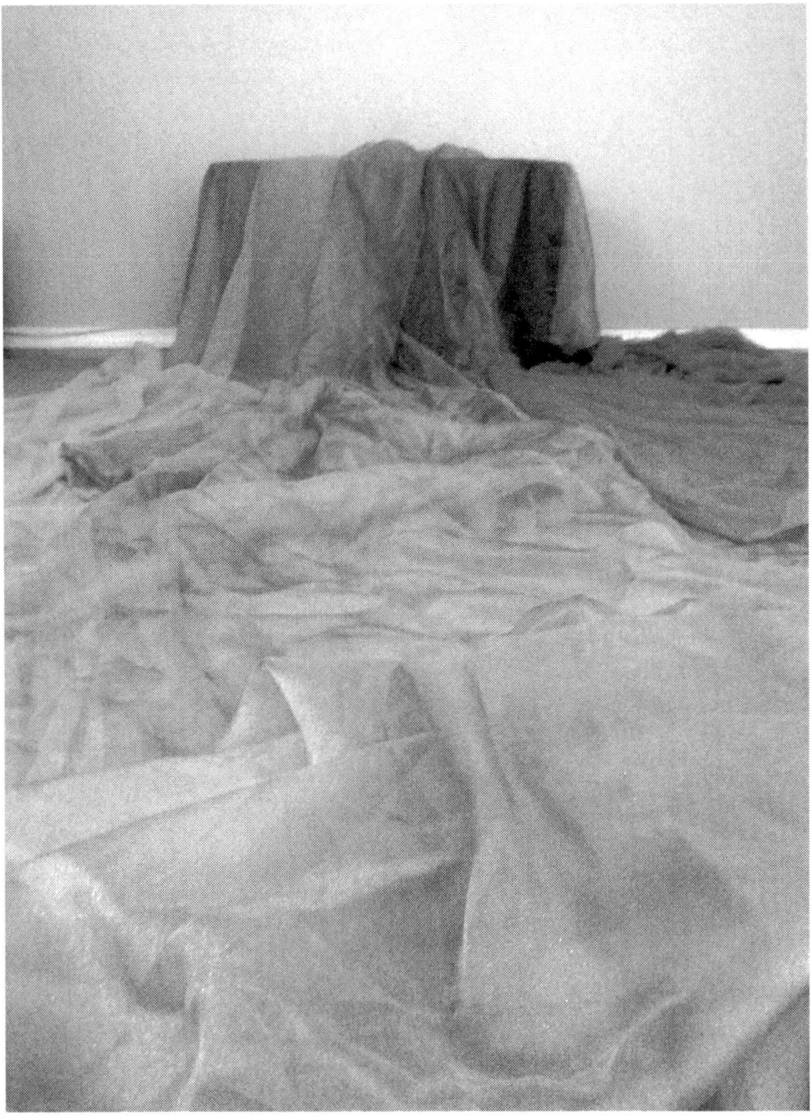

Figure 5.1 An example from the narradrama exercise of the Healing Mandala Room

Emotional Arousal through Externalization Work

The narradrama therapist will often work with the client on externalizing a problem through initially creating a visual aid, such as a mask, puppet, drawing, photo, or letter. The very act of creating the physical object "may directly access the social and emotional self, providing clients with opportunities to process emotions . . . If image making favors chance outcomes, [this] provides for an entryway to emotional expressivity" (Hass-Cohen and Findlay, 2015, p. 126). In addition to the possible emotional connectivity, the physical act of creating, and naming, their own preferred item helps clients separate themselves from the problem. From there, the therapist utilizes drama therapy techniques such as embodiment, interviewing, role reversal, and sculpting to assist the client in beginning to develop tools in order to change their relationship to the problem. This is often where the client experiences new and unexpected emotions and viewpoints about their initial problem, as their relationship to it has already begun to shift. Later on in the externalization work, the focus moves to processing and reflecting on the client's experience and revealed skills, which in turn can create new thoughts, behaviors, emotions, and preferred actions in relationship to their problem.

As an example, Emile, an ad executive in his late thirties, feels hopeless, self-critical, and defeated after being laid off from his agency. Early on in our sessions together, I ask him to create and name a mask of one of the problems that had been weighing heavily on him. He creates a mask, entitling it Imposter, which represents a strong, negative voice that repeatedly tells him he is not good enough. I then interviewed Imposter in order to discover moments when its successes faltered. This line of questioning, as it often does, revealed actions Emile had already taken, but was not consciously aware of, towards changing his relationship with Imposter. Since this exercise proved to be very powerful for him, he then creates a Personal Agency Mask, which he calls Truth, and which represents a preferred part of himself. Through a subsequent interview with Truth, Emile is able to further clarify tools he can use to positively change his relationship with Imposter. By bringing these new tools into the forefront, affirmative identity descriptions begin to grow.

In one particular session, a month later in therapy, Emile had a marked shift, as excerpted below, in a letter he writes to Imposter:

> "*It seems like you have always been in my head. Your voice led me to try to be better than others, to outdo my peers, to outdo you. I was told that hard work is the only thing that gets you anywhere, and that advice, combined with your voice, has led to years of not feeling like I will ever do enough to get to where I want to be. Until this month. These past several weeks of volunteering with at-risk youth really started to open my eyes to your lies. I couldn't save them and all my past hard work didn't help. It was showing up for them, and listening, and being okay with sharing myself with them that helped them. I finally began to realize: You are simply a problem that stalks the best of us. If I spent less time paying attention to you, you would probably move on. Because in reality: you are a coward. You are not*

*brave enough to be vulnerable and admit that life is not about being
something that one day you have arrived at, but about embracing my
resiliency, my intelligence, my humor, my skills, and admitting when
I am unsure."*

Novelty

Our brains seek out, and often quickly detect, novelty, or newness.
And it is by "exposing ourselves to new ideas and experiences" that we
experience novelty (Siegel, 2011, pp. 84–85). As "our brain searches for
patterns, it is alerted to change by its 'thirst' for novelty" (Tokuhama-
Espinosa, 2011, pp. 212). Novelty, however, is not the result of a single
cognitive process of neuronal activity, but the interplay of multiple cognitive processes and neural networks in which dopamine, which research
has found is an integral component in emotional processing, also plays a
critical role in this complex interaction (Chermahini & Hommel, 2010,
p. 458; Lhommée et al., 2014, p. 1).

Novelty through Creative Media and the Digital Space

Creative arts-based exercises and novelty go hand in hand, as the very
nature of creativity invites novelty. To illustrate, two narradrama-based
research studies, one a pilot and the second, a narrative inquiry, found
clients were successfully able to redefine and reconstruct themselves in
preferred ways through the following media-based exercises: 1) the Self
Commercial; and 2) the Personal Public Service Announcement (PPSA)
(Savage, 2015, pp. 50–150).

In the Self Commercial, which is videotaped and played back, the client creates a commercial where they, themselves, are the "product" that
they feel most represents them in a positive way. They then create a commercial where they advertise themselves as the "product" for sale. To
showcase an example from my own practice, Jordan, a 15-year-old who
has spent his adolescence in several group homes, chooses to advertise
himself as a "Zero Plus Five" energy drink, which thus created a new
vantage point in which to positively view himself as charismatic, full of
life, and able to motivate others.

The same result can also be seen in the PPSA, a novel exercise Savage
(2015, pp. 50–150) devised, in which clients create a mask and monologue
that represents their preferred self-identity—animating their masks with
a short monologue through the Morfo app on their tablets/smart phones.
In the last couple of years, I have often utilized creative arts-based apps as
they are a wonderful tool to aid in projecting clients' ideas, feelings, and
preferences due to the inherent immediacy of the digital space that allows
the client to be one click away from accessing the positive effects of a
digitally based exercise, which simultaneously can boost their probability

for memory consolidation (as discussed in detail in Chapter 2). Savage's app-based PPSA exercise is an ideal example of this. In my own practice, I have used a variation of this exercise, using an image-based app called WordPack, which transfers text into a text-based image. An example of this is used with Imani, an 18-year-old single parent, who creates the following preferred identity statement: "I hereby declare that I will be a role model to both myself and my daughter, to live a life that celebrates and respects all races, all sexual orientations, all women, all parents, and all people." Imani's statement, after typed into the WordPack app, becomes an image that she can then easily view after the session that day, and whenever and wherever she wishes.

A Careful Focus of Attention

The fourth area, a careful focus of attention, is a self-directed experience. A prime example of this is the utilization of mindfulness, which is "paying attention in a particular way; on purpose, in the present moment, and nonjudgmentally" (Kabat-Zinn, 1994, p. 4). This results in the focused attention that can "stimulate the neural firing in the brain" (Siegel, 2013, p. 116). Taking this concept into narradrama, mindful-based exercises that are centered around one or more art forms ensure that the client is able to draw their attention away from their problem state and into mindful awareness and presence that can "enable the brain to literally grow more integrative fibers that create [the client's] ability to regulate emotions, attention, thinking, and behavior" (Siegel, 2013, p. 116). Integrating mindfulness into my own work, one exercise I utilize often is a mindfulness pause, which I use after a significant enactment, sculpture, or interview; this is helpful for clients, during a reflection, to name how the dramatic moment registered, emotionally and bodily, during the pause.

A Careful Focus of Attention Using Mindfulness and Mandalas

The healing circle form of a mandala can be historically traced throughout many cultures, and according to Hass-Cohen and Findlay (2015), drawing a mandala invites a "concentrated mindfulness practice" and creates a "soothing and pleasurable" experience as the "intense concentration eases daily mind chatter" (pp. 341–342). For example, in the narradrama exercise of the Healing Mandala Room, a group session begins with a mindfulness meditation to find a tranquil place in their mind where individuals can notice their thoughts and feelings as they arise. From this place, group members then imagine healing images floating through them—taking notice of the color, texture, size, and sound of each one as they pass. At the end of the meditation, each group member chooses the image they most strongly connect to and then draw this image in a mandala to create a focal point before they move forward to actually creating a mandala room made out of fabrics. As an example, Mae, one of the members in an adult cancer support group class, creates her Mandala Room while listening to her favorite classical piece of music on her headphones. Her room is made of vibrant colored fabrics, some laid out on the floor mimicking that of ocean waves (Figure 5.1). When she enters the room, she dives into the fabric waves and laughs, rolling around and into each piece, as if she and the fabrics were one.

Victoria: A Case Example

Victoria, a programmer in her late thirties who has suffered from major depression, was recently released from an inpatient treatment program. I often start our sessions with a movement-based exercise, as she has expressed an affinity for dance, although she states that she lost her drive to dance some years ago. She often arrives with low energy and in what she calls her "over-thinking head," and the movement exercises immediately get her onto her feet and out of this state. As she has suffered from long bouts of depression in her life, it is imperative that she can begin to recognize more of her positive attributes and create space between herself and the depression. She begins by externalizing the role of what she names the Destroyer, describing this role as the critic who puts down all her attempts to live life the way she wants.

Early on in our sessions, she creates a mask of the Destroyer, which she paints in several layers of deep brown, folding in messily glued pieces of paper clips, sandpaper scraps, and crumpled up bits of paper. In a follow-up exercise, Victoria identifies a moment where the Destroyer overwhelms her, projecting this moment in the therapy space abstractly with chairs and fabrics. She sets up three chairs: she overturns the first chair, covering it with a black cloth, and then places the Destroyer mask on top of it. She leaves the second chair empty, in the middle of the room. Finally, on top of the third chair, she piles several pieces of dark fabric on top of each other. When done, Victoria leaves the space momentarily, before entering again to enact the moment in the environment she just created. When she re-enters, she drags her body towards the empty chair. Once there, she collapses onto it, blankly staring at the enormous pile of fabrics in front of her.

After a few moments, I walk over and sit beside her, in silence with her, taking in the scene. After a minute or so, I ask:

PD: Is this how you want the scene to be?
V: No.
PD: Well, what do you want it to be?
     Victoria gets up, walks over to the third chair, and attempts to grab the entire pile of fabrics in her arms. The pile is too large to hold, so she disperses the fabrics into smaller piles on the floor. She paces around, eying each pile.

PD: Is this how you want it to be?

After studying them for a bit, she starts pushing piles away with her foot towards the edges of the space, then creates even smaller piles, and pushes those away to the edge as well.

PD: What are these smaller piles?

V: Pieces of my depression.

She moves some of the small piles underneath the chairs, and studies the room.

PD: Is this how you want it?

V: Yes, I can manage this.

Victoria then pauses, before asking:

Could you take a picture of the scene? A picture of the little piles?

PD: Of course.

I take a photograph with a Polaroid I often utilize during session exercises and hand it to her. She holds the print in her hand, watching it as it develops. When the image appears, she looks up at me, proclaiming:

V: There, now they don't have any power.

After working with Victoria over several sessions, she starts to become more aware of her positive attributes. She creates a mask of a preferred role, which she names Ariel, describing it as an inner guide. Some sessions, as is expected, feeling the weight of the Destroyer, she enters therapy withdrawn and quiet. The beginning of the following session is one of those times:

Beginning to move around the space, I say:

PD: Victoria, walk with me.

V: (*looking down at her lap*) Oh. I don't know. Maybe not today.

PD: Just try it.

V: Uh, ok. (*She starts to slowly walk towards me*)

PD: That's it. So, have you discovered anything new this week?

V: I don't know.

PD: Did you think any more about Ariel?

V: Sometimes.

PD: What about becoming Ariel for a few minutes?

V: I don't feel her . . . It's hard to find her. Especially when I'm feeling like this.

PD: Like what?

V: You know. Down. Like crap.

PD: Would you like her to find you?

V: I don't know. Sure.

PD: Why don't you use your Ariel mask? Maybe that could help.

Victoria goes over to pick up the mask, puts it on, and returns to walk alongside me again.

PD: Ariel, Victoria tells me it is hard to find you.

V: It isn't hard usually. But she can't find me when she's in a funk.

PD: What would you say to Victoria?

V: (*After a long pause, she says*) Well, Victoria, you need to keep moving. (*She picks up the pace*). YES, keep moving! Don't stay in bed. Keep active; it makes you feel better. Stretch and move around. Like this.
      Victoria, as Ariel, runs in place.

V: That's right! Destroyer is trying to take over! You need to stop worrying. Always worrying. Look up at the sky. Take a breath. Remind yourself that you have strength inside of you. You can move forward into a future that you want, and you can be everything that you want to be!
      Victoria comes to a halt, takes a deep breath, and takes off her mask.

V: Whoa, she exhales. That was crazy.

PD: What do you mean?

V: I just really surprised myself. I mean, I can really see and feel all my passion and energy right now. (*Victoria appears flushed and exhilarated*)

During a session near the end of her therapy, we discuss some of her new life practices and how they help her with stress at work. I invite her to show me a scene of what it looks like to come home from such a day.

Victoria sets up a scene in her living room using the existing furniture and fabrics in the therapy space: a small couch, two chairs, and a large plastic bin overflowing with fabrics. When she enters the scene to begin her enactment, Victoria pantomimes shutting the door behind her followed by a long exhale before nearly collapsing onto the couch. Once there for a few moments, she gets up and starts moving around the room until she spots her journal popping out of her bag. She focuses on it for a moment before taking a long breath and closing her eyes.

When she opens them again, she takes note of the chest of fabrics, then goes over to it, and pulls out a long yellow cotton piece, holding it close to her chest. Next, she chooses bright purple chiffon, forming it into a ball, before she rolls it across the room. Then she reaches into her pocket, taking out her phone. Scrolling on the screen, she locates her favorite song and hits play, ensuring the volume in all the way up.

Victoria begins humming, but as the song continues to pick up in tempo, her voice picks up volume, now singing louder, belting it with all of her voice, until—reaching the chorus—she spontaneously jumps up from the floor. She runs to the fabrics, singing, grabbing as much fabric in her arms as she can before beginning to dance, fabrics full in her arms. Finally, the song nearing an end, she is out of breath, but exhilarated. While singing the last line, she throws all the fabrics up into the air during her final note. Grinning, she watches them fly on their way back down, before joining them to rest in a heap of color on the ground.

As is evident from the above three examples, over the course of our work together, Victoria makes a sea-change shift from despondent to hopeful to triumphant. From the "aha" moment, where she is overcome with an energy and emotion that fills her body, breath, and words, to successfully re-defining herself and her relationship to depression, Victoria and the neuroscience-informed work explored in her sessions is a testament to the integrated connectivity and transformative power of the arts, therapy, and brain science.

Conclusion

As I think back to that conference five years ago where I first heard Siegel speak, I marvel at how much my therapeutic practice has deepened as a result of implementing what I have learned through interpersonal neurobiology and affective neuroscience. Siegel's four conditions have since been well integrated into my work, both with clients and as an instructor in my field. Not only is the importance of arousing positive emotions folded into my work, but I continue to strive to find new ways for my clients and students to experience the benefits of the integration of mindfulness, positive emotions, and the creative arts therapies. As research in the field grows, my knowledge will continue to expand and fuel my work. It is my hope that my clients, through experiencing sustained change and growth on a physiological and psychological level, will be equipped to move forward to a new life path that honors and celebrates their uniqueness.

Notes

1. Neurogenesis is the process by which neurons are generated from neuro stem cells. This happens, along with synapse formation and myelin growth, and can take place in response to experiences throughout our life (Siegel, 2011, p. 4).
2. Alexis, along with all other client examples used in this chapter, are composites.

References

Beaudoin, M.-N., & Zimmerman, J. (2011). Narrative therapy & interpersonal neurobiology: Revisiting classic practices, developing new emphases. *Journal of Systemic Therapies*, *30*(1), 1–13.

Chermahini, S. A., & Hommel, B. (2010). The (b)link between creativity and dopamine: Spontaneous eye blink rate predict and dissociate divergent and convergent thinking. *Cognition*, *115*, 458–465.

Cozolino, L. (2016). *Why therapy works*. New York, NY: W. W. Norton & Company Inc.

Hass-Cohen, N., & Findlay, J. C. (2015). *Art therapy & the neuroscience of relationships, creativity, & resiliency*. New York, NY: W. W. Norton & Company Inc.

Kabat-Zinn, J. (1994). *Wherever you go there you are*. New York, NY: Hyperion.

Landy, R. J. (2008). *The couch & the stage*. New York, NY: Jason Aronson.

Lhommée, E., Batir, A., Quesada, J. L., Aardouin, C., Fraix, V., Seigneuret, E., Chabardés, S., Benabid, A. L., Pollack, P., & Krack, P. (2014). Dopamine and the biology of creativity: Lessons from Parkinson's disease. *Frontiers in Neurology, 5:55*(11), 1–11.

Morfo. (2013). SunSpark Labs (Version 2.2.1), [Mobile application software]. Retrieved from http://www.morfoapp.com

Savage, M. (2015). *Making personal public service announcements with adopted young women from foster care: A narrative inquiry.* (Doctoral Dissertation). Lesley University, Boston, MA. (204 pp.; #3706869).

Siegel, D. (2011). *Mindsight.* New York, NY: Random House.

Siegel, D. (2013). *Brainstorm.* New York, NY: Jeremy P. Tarcher.

Tokuhama-Espinosa, T. (2011). *Mind, brain & education science: A comprehensive guide to the new brain-based teaching.* New York, NY: W. W. Norton & Company Inc.

WordPack. (2013). A. Tataurov (Version 1.1), [Mobile application software]. Retrieved from http://itunes.apple.com

6 Tapping into the Power of the Brain-Heart-Gut Axis

Addressing Embodied Aspects of Intense Emotions such as Anxiety

Marie-Nathalie Beaudoin

Introduction

Brain research has highlighted the crucial role of emotions in shaping the brain's activity and individuals' responses to life (Damasio, 2000). In particular, as summarized in Chapter 2 of this book, emotions coined as negative reduce the blood flow to the frontal lobe and narrow attention, while emotions considered positive are associated with increased mental and regulatory capacities.

Intense emotions manifest themselves through a number of physiological markers throughout the body (Ekman, 2007). Anxiety for example, often accelerates the heart, shifts the lungs into taking shallower in-breaths, immobilizes digestion, and increases blood flow to the legs (to run away from saber-toothed tigers). Facial muscles, including the jaw, become tenser and eyes tend to blink more frequently (Harrigan & O'Connel, 1996). The amygdala in the limbic system fires furiously to arouse certain areas of the brain, and de-activate others, such as those associated with connection and relationships.

Until recently, clinical work in post-modern collaborative therapies privileged therapeutic explorations of cognitive, affective, behavioral, relational, contextual and personal (identity) aspects of experience. The advent of new research on vertical integration (Siegel, 2012) has highlighted the importance of examining embodied experiences—that is, the various body sensations associated with problematic and preferred experiences of oneself (Beaudoin, 2015; Beaudoin & Zimmerman, 2011). Metaphorically, failure to examine salient aspects of embodied states can be akin to inferring the full image of a puzzle by looking only at a few pieces. Knowledge of the remaining embodied information can provide key clinical material, and certain organs can act as doorways in and out of certain states (Beaudoin, 2015). This is particularly the case with organs containing neuron cells such as the brain (100,000 billion), heart (40,000) and gut (500 million) (Furness, 2006; Pereira, Cerqueira, Palha, & Sousa, 2013; Van Der Wall & Van Der Gilst, 2012). Neuron cells have the neuroplastic ability to learn and are therefore particularly vulnerable to being shaped by experience. Clients seeking assistance with intense problematic emotions typically struggle with associated intense physiological reactions involving the brain, heart and gut. This is visible when working with people struggling with anxiety, stress and panic attacks, whose minds and bodies have developed habitual ways of responding rapidly and hugely to certain stimulus. Through the process of interoception (Wiens, 2005), clients are often aware that these reactions are excessive but feel that their body is out of control.

This was the case for Cathy, a 33-year-old nurse, who had successfully worked with me when she was in nursing school, in her early twenties. She was then struggling with panic attacks and a sense of overwhelm in her life, in particular about working in medical emergency settings. In those days, anxiety led her to worry about making mistakes, and left her overanalyzing everything she did during and after the fact. Our work had helped her connect with her preferred identity, a sense of self as being capable, knowledgeable and compassionate, which she owed to a loving aunt. We had also explored some basic mindfulness meditation practices that she then diligently practiced every day. Cathy now re-contacts me and schedules an appointment to discuss a recent wave of anxiety-producing experiences.

The purpose of this chapter is to render visible the value of embodied conversations, an emerging path in collaborative therapies. Segments of the therapeutic conversation that takes place with Cathy will be examined along with relevant research on the brain, heart and gut, which justifies certain clinical directions. At any given point in a therapeutic conversation, therapists make choices based on a client's experience at that moment, context, therapist's knowledge and understandings, historical data on the problem, preferences and therapeutic journey. Conversational crossroads are explicitly acknowledged here to highlight different directions without elevating one over the other. This comparison between current embodied work, and how the therapeutic conversation would have proceeded before my exposure to interpersonal neurobiology in the early 2000, explains why one option might be better suited to the current consultation.

Understanding the Embodied Problem

C: *Since I last saw you, I've done quite well with managing my anxiety and I'm actually happy with my nursing job now (. . .). The reason I wanted to talk today is that my co-workers are trying to set me up with dates. I'm open to it, but it triggers so much anxiety every time, that sometimes I wonder if it's even worth it.*

MN: *So you're open to the idea of dating but the anxiety makes you wonder if it's worth it? How does the anxiety affect you more specifically?*

C: *Well, it makes me anticipate and be nervous the whole day prior to the date. My day is wasted in this mental torture. I go back and forth between wanting to cancel, and then not being able to actually pick up my phone and text him. I've never actually canceled so far and made myself go because it would be nice to have a partner, but then I'm also awkward during the date.*

The early stage of this clinical conversation starts with the usual orientation to the presenting issue. It can be helpful to ask a few general questions before moving to specific details, as this loitering often orients the therapist, sheds light on what the client has already observed about the problem and is fertile ground for the development of a tentative experience-near externalization and for collecting information on efforts and successes. In Cathy's situation, the sequence of event usually involved her co-worker telling her about an interesting young man and getting Cathy's permission to give him her phone number. He would then call or text and, as soon as a specific date was scheduled, usually a dinner, anxiety would start eroding her excitement, with the worst of it being just before or during the event. Cathy had endured in this way, meeting three separate men, and felt stuck with anxiety always stalking her and the inability to fully be her preferred self. I inquire about how she has continued to attend these dates in spite of anxiety's torture and she acknowledges that scheduling them on weekdays, after busy workdays, prevents the agonizing waiting time. She is then only left with the anxiety during the event, which she controls by intently immersing herself in others' experiences so that there is no room for anxiety's voice. This way of being, which we uncovered over a decade ago, has worked well for her until now. Since the old strategy is less effective in this recent adventure, I invite her to share a specific example of the new challenge to examine novel or previously unnoticed aspects of the problem. I am careful to elicit *felt* territories of experience rather than dwelling in intellectual exchanges *about* her experience. Reactivating vivid lived experience in the therapy room offers three main benefits (Beaudoin, 2013): 1. It provides a more complex understanding of the various facets of the problem; 2. It creates an opportunity to craft strategies from within physiological arousal which can more thoroughly neutralize problem experiences; 3. It strengthens regulating neural networks in the brain by weaving connections between vivid experiences and a supportive observing process. As mentioned earlier, if embodied emotions are part of the problem, embodied emotions have to be part of the solution. Seeking vivid experiences is helpful as long as therapists avoid re-traumatizing or re-overwhelming clients, and therefore ensure that the physiological activation remains within the borders of people's ability to regulate their experience (see Siegel's window of tolerance).

MN: *Can you give me a recent example of a dating-related moment when the anxiety might have affected you?*

Cathy: *Yes, two weekends ago, I was going to meet a gentleman who appeared to have a lot in common with me. As I was driving to the restaurant, anxiety kept on torturing me with "What if I like him? What if I don't like him? What if I get sick? What if I have nausea? What if I throw up in front of him?"*

The conversation continues with a list of all the "what ifs" triggered by anxiety and are ultimately organized in two themes: the implication of liking or not the prospective boyfriend, and the worries about becoming sick during the date. Since Cathy stated that the second was the utmost worst, even though she had not thrown up since childhood, the remaining conversation focused on the worry of getting sick. Many directions are possible here, but with the new research on the importance of bodily states, I chose to explore a moment at a restaurant when anxiety made its appearance and triggered a sensation of being sick.

Cathy: I was really enjoying his story and when the server interrupted him to ask a question, I thought, "Wow, this is going so well! I'm relaxed, talking naturally and even joking!" And then, out of the blue I felt a huge wave of anxiety and nausea, like I was going to be sick right there and then, it horrified me.

Actual embodied questions	Hypothetical disembodied questions
MN: So you were noticing that you were relaxed and enjoying yourself, and suddenly the anxiety infiltrated that observation process? (Yeah!) What did your attention focus on more specifically? What happened to your body in that split second of observing? Where in your body did the anxiety grab you the most?	*MN: So it felt like this huge wave of nausea took over, out of the blue. Let's start by examining how you were managing the anxiety before that happened and how you were succeeding in enjoying this dinner (. . .). Then, what did the anxiety get you to think in that split second? Were you able to recover from this assault? What were the micro-steps involved in this recovery?*
These questions attempt to include an enhanced awareness of the physiological reactions that dominate her experience. I'm wondering if anxiety takes advantage of the observing process to infiltrate her embodied experience of herself.	These questions could have been productive as long as they eventually got to physical sensations. Answers might have included: "To focus on him, and force myself to be immersed in his story"; "To worry about being sick." The third question could have led to more richly described, but known, strategies.

Recent studies in brain research have highlighted that people struggling with anxiety generally show one and/or two different patterns of brain activation (Engels et al., 2007): 1. The problem is mostly triggered and sustained by cognitions and worries, a process dominated by the left brain; or 2. The problem is triggered by bodily changes which can *precede* conscious registration of an emotion in the brain. The later process is mostly associated with right brain activation and in many instances, involves skewed reactions from the heart and/or gut brain.

Cathy: *Hum . . . I think I checked whether my stomach was all right and then I discovered that I was actually NOT doing well. I thought "Oh my gosh! I'm not well after all, what do I do? I really AM nervous, can he tell? What if this nausea doesn't go away?"*

MN: *So anxiety made you check your stomach, and right after that, all of a sudden, you didn't feel good. Is it possible that the anxiety itself made your stomach feel sick?*

Cathy: *Yeah, now that I think of it, I'm pretty sure it did, because I was fine before.*

MN: *How does the anxiety convince you to check if your stomach is alright?*

Cathy: *Well, if I check ahead before being sick then I might be able to avoid being sick in front of him.*

Anxiety gets most people to surveil that which they fear the most. It gets people to track, anticipate and respond intensely to interoceptive perceptions which amplify a sense of "danger" and inadvertently create a self-perpetuating feedback loop (Paulus & Stein, 2010). When the object of worry is a physiological activation, the very process of checking on a problem, in an anxiety-conducive context, can itself activate the sympathetic nervous system. As such, people who worry about blood pressure or asthma may find themselves activating these problems when simply checking on their status. Since strong emotions, meaning, relevance and repetition are powerful brain encoders (Beaudoin, 2010), several instances of this co-activation (cognitive checking + physiological arousal) can wire strong neural networks that are triggered easily and quickly.

In the next exchange with Cathy, we briefly take apart this belief by first reactivating the sensations portion of the memory of the event. Memories are not videotapes but rather reconstruction of events (Ecker, Ticic, & Hulley, 2012), and just as puzzles, it is often easier to reconstruct them by starting with the retrieval of peripheral information such as body posture and sensations (Beaudoin, 2010).

Actual embodied questions	Hypothetical disembodied questions
MN: Can you close your eyes for a second and go back to that moment, remembering yourself sitting in the chair, in the restaurant? What kind of sensations did the anxiety create in your stomach?	*So did the anxiety trick you into thinking that checking will be helpful and prevent problems, when in reality it opens the door to more of itself? Does it sabotage your enjoyment? What is that about?*

Cathy: *A sense of dread and tightness. Like all its content where moving as in a blender out of control.*

MN: *So a sense of dread, tightness, a blender out of control, anything else?*

Cathy: *I felt dizzy too, as if the world was turning around me suddenly.*

MN: *So you were dizzy and the world was turning. How were you breathing? Did it also affect your heart?*

Cathy (whitish, still eyes closed):   *I wasn't daring to breath, I didn't want to add any movement down there, I didn't want to risk allowing the dinner to come up, I was holding my breath, I guess you could say I was breathing in a shallow way, trying to control it, and my heart was beating too fast in my chest.*

MN: *You didn't dare to breath and your heart was beating fast. So would you say you were sort of captured by the anxiety and its focus on your chest and abdomen? (Yeah). I wonder if the very action of observing your stomach opens the door to anxiety?*

Cathy (opening her eyes):   *Yeah . . . it's probably anxiety's headquarter.*

We eventually conclude that her body would just "tell her" if she was sick, she doesn't "need" anxiety to check it and act as a messenger since it seems to distort the information. Anxiety has a strong hold on Cathy's body, enough to trigger intense physical sensations that then escalate almost beyond her control. If the problem's hold on her experience comes from her stomach and gut, then the "solution" must take into account her stomach and gut. This is particularly true given that messages from the gut *to* the brain are faster than the other way around (Mayer, 2011). This partly explains why the alarming sensations very suddenly flood her experience. In fact, recent research suggests that 90% of the communication between the brain and gut consists of the gut sending information *to* the brain through the vagus nerve (Hadhazy, 2010). In Cathy's situation, we can speculate that the gut itself has developed skewed neural networks that send a signal of alarm as soon as she is in an anxiety-provoking situation *and* focuses her attention on possible sensations in her abdomen. This skewed program needs to be retrained as a muscle which has taken the habit of spasming during a specific movement. Cathy agrees that trusting her body to inform her in its own time, rather than allowing anxiety to go check there, might help. As discussed in Chapter 3, the very act of naming problems and process has also been found to facilitate regulation. Metaphorically, it can be said that the frontal lobe is in a better position to manage a problem, and access its "solutions," when problematic and preferred experiences are identified and labeled. As coined by Siegel and mentioned elsewhere in this book, "to name it is to tame it."

The conversation then proceeds to examining preferred-embodied experiences by discussing how the evening evolved after that moment of anxiety and panic.

Examining Preferred-Embodied Experiences

MN: *How did you attempt to recover from anxiety's grip on your abdomen?*

Cathy: *I told myself to focus on him, on his story, to ignore my body. I also found an escape route, I told myself: "if there's a problem I can say I've got to go, and run to the restroom."*

MN: *You found an escape route, and focused on him. Did you ever reconnect with enjoying the evening?*

Cathy (laughing):   *Yeah, because an old friend from college walked in unexpectedly and distracted me. But I can't count on that happening every time!*

Actual embodied questions	Hypothetical disembodied questions
MN (smiling): *So checking in with your body leaves you vulnerable to being kidnapped by anxiety and the main way out right now is to focus on other people? (Yeah!) Now going back to when you were enjoying yourself, talking to the unexpected friend who walked in, how might you describe the sensations in your abdomen and chest then?* Cathy: *Hum . . . I don't know . . . there aren't any.*	*Let's examine what happened when you were distracted by the college friend. What did you focus on when you took control of the anxiety?* This can be a valuable direction and we had actually journeyed on this path in the past, which, again, is how this empathic client successfully manages many anxiety-provoking situations. Given past knowledge of this client, there is a great likelihood she would have answered, "focusing on the old friend." This direction is not as viscerally embodied as the other, and therefore not sufficient in the face of intense challenges.

Articulating sensations associated with her preferred experiences of her body can provide more power to Cathy's growing sense of agency. Sometimes the effort to ignore an experience requires an enormous amount of energy that may be put to better use by fueling preferred experiences instead. Research shows that once intense physiological reactions associated with "negative" emotions are triggered, it is difficult to use top-down cognitive processes to regulate bottom-up experiences (Engels et al., 2010). In other words, *controlling intense emotions with reason alone has limited effectiveness*. It is more helpful to assist clients in *replacing* an intense physiological reaction with another, rather than cognitively attempting to stop it. This can be accomplished by developing expertise in embodied preferred experiences that, in and of themselves, will be associated with alternative ways of thinking.

In Cathy's situation, as with many other clients, there is an acute awareness of problem-related sensations and a reduced awareness of preferred-embodied sensations. This leaves clients fighting an emotion with reason and *sensing* the problem-related, but not the desirable, physiological activation. Careful scaffolding and memory work has to be instigated to help clients tap into these sensations, as demonstrated below:

MN: *If you close your eyes and go back to the restaurant, talking to your college friend, which area of your body stands out as being involved in this relaxed enjoyment?*

Cathy: *Hum . . . maybe my face . . . it's been pretty easy to get my face to smile and fake it until I make it.*

MN: *So your smile can fake it until you make it, can you say more about that?*

Cathy: *Anxiety has rarely touched my smile. Everyone can see my face so I've become really good at always hiding the anxiety.*

MN: *If anxiety can rarely touch your smile, would you say that your face is in some way an area where you're in control, like* **your** *headquarter?*

Cathy (Pleased):   *Yeah! I like that idea! Smiling can be my "control headquarter"!*

MN: *Can you say more about the sensations in your face when you're in control and smiling?*

There are 42 muscles in the face, and smiling has been found to mobilize up to 12 of those depending on whether the smile is genuine or not. Facial muscle contraction has been found to affect the brain's regulation of emotions (Laird & Lacasse, 2014). This phenomenon was initially discovered in "botulinum toxin (BTX) induced facial muscle paralysis," where subjects exposed to emotional stimuli reported less intense emotional experiences than average because their facial muscles were immobilized, therefore limiting the expected brain activity usually associated with that specific emotion (Keillor, Barret, Crucian, Kortenkamp, & Heilman, 2002). The brain essentially likes to be congruent with the body, so if facial muscles are not expressing an emotion, the brain will limit its inner experience of that emotion. The mind-body relationship is bidirectional and reciprocal (Herbert & Pollatos, 2012). In other words, while we all knew that happiness made us smile, research has also shown that smiling can make the brain state of happiness more accessible (Critchley & Nagai, 2012; Davis, Senghas, & Ochsner, 2009). As a result, cultivating embodied positive emotions intrinsically provides an anxiety countervailing state by: 1. limiting the intensity of a negative emotion such as anxiety; 2. triggering a physiological upward spiral (Garland et al., 2010); and 3. enhancing the production of dopamine, a neurotransmitter associated with satisfaction and happiness.

Cathy (thinking): *Hum . . . Let me see . . . My eyes feel bright . . . I smile . . . my forehead and eyebrows are not all crunched up . . . my jaw is more relaxed and I'm talkative; and I guess I move my hands more when I talk.*

MN: *So your hands are involved too in the state of being more relaxed and in control. What might they do?*

Cathy: *I might put my hand on the other person's shoulder to show I'm paying attention or play with something . . . my hands sort of come alive. They're moving of their own mind.*

MN: *If there was an image or a metaphor that could capture how you are being in control of your face, your smile and your hands, what might it be?*

Cathy (thinking): *I'm . . . uh . . . like a puppet master!*

MN (intrigued): *So you're like a puppet master?! Can you say more?*

Cathy: *Well, when I'm in control, the puppet master is sort of the one who pulls the strings on different parts of my body, decides what people see and what I do!*

MN: *Might the puppet master be helpful in preventing an anxiety attack and keeping you away from anxiety's headquarter?*

Cathy (excitedly): *Oh! I see! When I want to check how things are going, I can direct the strings of my puppet to my face and hands . . . and that means noticing that I'm feeling in control! Like I'm checking if I'm in control of my hands and face instead of my stomach! Wow! Now I have a picture of me in control! I didn't know I had a silent co-driver that's adjusting where I'm going without anxiety knowing! Cool!*

MN: *You had a silent co-driver!?*

Cathy (very excited): *Yeah! I guess this means that the puppet master is more powerful than the anxiety and I never gave it credit!*

Actual embodied questions	Hypothetical disembodied questions
MN: *Can you give me another example of a time when the puppet master might have been a silent co-driver and taken control, using your face and hands to help you deal with anxiety?*	MN: *Who might have inspired this puppet master and silent co-driver? Is there anyone you know who might have one too?* This question could be really helpful, but in the context of attempting to increase this client's control over intense physiological reactions, it may be more helpful to continue exploring her experience of her body at this time.

Cathy: *Yes, as a matter of fact, now I see that I have been using this occasionally without realizing it! I did it on Halloween too, when my roommates wanted to go out and anxiety got me all nervous about it. Now I can do this more!*

The conversation continues and extracts more details about the physiological sensations associated with being in control and enjoying herself. Cathy progressively articulates that she manages to not feel the anxiety, to freeze it, and replaces it with excitement. Because of the mood congruent recall phenomena (also coined State Dependent Recall) (Matt, Vazquez, & Campbell, 1992), where the brain more readily remembers memories encoded in similar states, this fuels the recollection of another successful event, a book club meeting she organized at her home. This time the conversation focuses on examining the general sensations associated with her chest and abdomen. She discovers that, at her best, her chest feels like a balloon filled with excitement, her breathing is slower, and her gut is invisible, as if it was a light switch in an "off" position. When prompted for details, she explains that her abdomen feels empty, solid, not moving inside and quiet. I invite her to also describe her heart since, again, the heart contains an important set of neural networks often recruited in intense emotions.

MN: *So your abdomen feels quiet, empty, solid, not moving. How about your heart? Can you close your eyes, go back to that moment, and see if you can describe the sensations in your heart in more details?*

Cathy: *Hum . . . Well it's beating a little faster as a background drum in an orchestra but not taking over and dominating, just contributing to the excitement.*

Research has shown that a coherent heart rate variability (HRV), where the sympathetic and parasympathetic nervous system function in harmony, optimizes brain functioning (Thayer, Hansen, Saus-Rose, & Johnson, 2009). Such coherence is typically experienced during positive emotions and can be associated with a phenomena of brain and gut entrainment (Van Der Wall & Van Der Gilst, 2012). In other words, important neural areas of the body (such as the brain, the heart and the gut) can each act as doorway into embodied preferred selves (Beaudoin, 2015). Exploring experiences of these organs during successful moments of self-control provides clients with:

- increased awareness of embodied preferred selves;
- strong and preferred neural networks in various location of the body; and
- multiple ways of entering desirable brain states.

We have now collected a series of observations about her body in both the problem and preferred state. Her newfound knowledge of embodied ways of being affords her more choices when faced with a challenging event— that is, refocusing her attention to interoceptive experiences associated with control provided Cathy with a powerful option to counteract anxiety.

References

Beaudoin, M.-N. (2010). *The SKiLL-ionaire in every child: Boosting children's socio-emotional skills using the latest in brain research*. San Francisco, CA: Goshawk Publications.

Beaudoin, M.-N. (2013). *Neurobiology and narrative therapy: Making changes stick in everyday lives*. San Diego, CA: Alexander Street Press Videos.

Beaudoin, M.-N. (2015). Flourishing with positive emotions: Increasing clients' repertoire of problem counter-state. *Journal of Systemic Therapies, 34*(2), 1–12.

Beaudoin, M.-N., & Zimmerman, J. (2011). Narrative therapy and interpersonal neurobiology: Revisiting classic practices, developing new emphases. *Journal of Systemic Therapies, 48*(1), 1–13.

Critchley, H., & Nagai, Y. (2012). How emotions are shaped by bodily states. *Emotion Review, 4*(2), 163–168.

Damasio, A. (2000). *The feeling of what happens: Body and emotions in the making of consciousness*. New York, NY: Mariner.

Davis, J., Senghas, A., & Ochsner, K. N. (2009). How does facial feedback modulate emotional experience? *Journal of Research & Personality, 43*(5), 822–829.

Ecker, B., Ticic, R., & Hulley, L. (2012). *Unlocking the emotional brain: Eliminating symptoms at their roots using memory reconsolidation*. New York, NY: Routledge.

Ekman, P. (2007). *Emotions revealed* (2nd ed.). New York, NY: Holt.

Engels, A., Heller, W., Mohanty, A., Herrington, J., Banish, M. T., Webb, A. G., & Miller, J. A. (2007). Specificity of regional brain activity in anxiety types during emotional processing. *Psychophysiology, 44*(3), 352–363.

Engels, A., Heller, W., Spielberg, J., Warren, S., Sutter, P., Banish, M., & Miller, G. (2010). Co-occurring anxiety affects patterns of brain activity in depression. *Cognitive, Affective and Behavioral Neuroscience, 10*(1), 141–156.

Furness, J. B. (2006). *The Enteric Nervous System*. Blackwell, Oxford, p. 274.

Garland, E. L., Fredrickson, B., Kring, A. M., Johnson, D. P., Meyers, P. S., & Penn, D. L., (2010). Upward spirals of positive emotions counter downward spiral of negativity: Insights from the broaden-and-build theory and affective neuroscience on the treatment of emotion dysfunction and deficits in psychopathology. *Clinical Psychology Review, 30*(7), 849–864.

Hadhazy, A. (2010, February 12). Think twice: How the gut's second brain influences mood and well-being. *Scientific American (www.scientificamerican.com)*.

Harrigan, J., & O'Connell, D. (1996). Facial movements during anxiety states. *Personality and Individual Differences, 21*, 205–212.

Herbert, B. M., & Pollatos, O. (2012). The body in the mind: On the relationship between interoception and embodiement. *Topics in Cognitive Science, 4*(4), 692–704.

Keillor, J. M., Barret, A. M., Crucian, J. P., Kortenkamp, S., & Heilman, K. M. (2002). Emotional experience and perception in the absence of facial feedback. *Journal of the International Neuropsychology Society, 8*, 130–135.

Laird, J., & Lacasse, K. (2014). Bodily influence on emotional feelings accumulating evidence and extensions of William Jame's theory of emotion. *Emotion Review, 6*(1), 27–34.

Matt, G., Vazquez, C., & Campbell, W. K. (1992). Mood congruent recall of affectively toned stimuli: A meta-analytic review. *Clinical Psychology Review, 12*, 225–257.

Mayer, E. (2011). Gut feeling: The emerging biology of gut-brain communication. *National Review of Neuroscience, 12*(8), 1038–1043.

Paulus, M. P., & Stein, M. B. (2010). Interoception in anxiety and depression. *Brain Structure & Function, 214*(5–6), 451–463.

Pereira, V. H., Cerqueira, J. J., Palha, J. A., Sousa, N. (2014). Stressed brain, diseased heart: a review on the pathophysiologic mechanisms of neurocardiology. *International Journal of Cardiology, 166*: 30–37.

Siegel, D. (2012). *The developing mind: How relationships and the brain interact to shape who we are* (2nd ed.). New York, NY: Guilford Press.

Thayer, J. F., Hansen, A., Saus-Rose, E., & Johnson, B. (2009). Heart rate variability, prefrontal neural functions, and cognitive performance: The neurovisceral integration perspective on self-regulation, adaptation and health. *Annals of Behavioural Medicine, 37*, 141–153.

Van Der Wall, E. E., & Van Der Gilst, W. H. (2012). Neurocardiology: Close interaction between heart and brain. *Netherland Heart Journal, 10*, 1–6.

Wiens, S. (2005). Interoception in emotional experience. *Current Opinion in Neurology, 18*(4), 442–447.

7 Narrative Neurotherapy (NNT)
Scaffolding Identity States

Jan Ewing, Ron Estes, and Brandon Like

Introduction

How do narratives shape our physiology and experience of the world? How do acts of interpretation shape our actions, bodies, identities, and experiences of life? Are there ways to intentionally interpret and construct narratives that shape our physiology? How might we learn to develop and sustain the narrative interpretations that allow us to inhabit the identities we prefer? These questions have influenced our work to emphasize the relationship between narratives and physiology. We refer to these expanding practices as Narrative Neurotherapy (NNT).

Contemporary neurophysiological research contributes new ways of thinking and speaking about psychotherapy. Consider neuroplasticity, or the brain's ability to change both functional and structural qualities through new experiences. Neuroplasticity represents the basis of learning, and has led some to suggest that psychotherapy is a learning process where improvement emerges through the physiological rewiring of neural networks (Grawe, 2007; LeDoux, 2002). To think of psychotherapy as learning represents a distinct shift from the metaphor of psychotherapy as healing. Therapy might be measured through improved relationships with others, increased self-regulation when confronted with challenges, thinking differently about situations accompanied with a sense of agency or purpose, or even noticing changes in physical sensations and a reduction of symptoms. Interestingly, these benefits are not always associated with neurophysiological processes, even though they rely upon them.

Narrative Scaffolding and Neuroscience

Michael White (2007) introduced the idea of scaffolding conversations adapted from work on social learning initiated by Lev Vygotsky (1962) and Jerome Bruner (Wood, Bruner, & Ross, 1976). White noted the constraining effects of culture and daily habits on people's lives, and considered social learning theory as a way to assist people to formulate new ideas and identities in response to challenges. Vygotsky and Bruner realized that most learning occurs in collaborative social interactions. The space in which learning emerges came to be known as the *Zone of Proximal Development* (Vygotsky, 1978), where a person moves from *what is known* to *what could be known* through a progression supported by others. Knowledge and skills are scaffolded into more complex formulations through conversations. Michael White used these scaffolding conversations to support people moving from *problem-saturated stories* to expanded re-tellings better aligned with their emerging *preferred identities* (White, 2007).

Inhabiting Our Lives: Learning and Biased Neural Networks

The growth and connectivity of neurons is the basic mechanism of learning and adaptation. Learning can be understood as neural changes in a number of ways, including shifts in the connectivity between neurons and the growth of new neurons. These are examples of neural plasticity, or the ability of the nervous system to change in response to experience (Bailey, Bartsch, & Kandel, 1996; Hebb, 1949; Paulsen & Sejnowski, 2000). Experience and learning cause structural and functional shifts throughout the brain (Kozorovitskiy, Gross, & Kopil, 2005), leading to the creation and maintenance of biased neural networks. Through repeated patterns of synchronous activity, groups of neurons become more likely to activate together in response to a stimulus. Individual neurons grow denser connections, become more sensitive to neurotransmitter chemical messengers, or develop myelinated connections that facilitate rapid signal propagation when activated (Gluck, Mercado, & Myers, 2008).

Biased networks of brain activity shape perception/interpretation and behavior. When our constructed identities and physiologies converge, we are *inhabiting* our lives. Biased neural networks are related to both the habits of daily life and symptoms of a mental health diagnosis. The biases of neural networks are necessary: without them we would not be able to learn new information, remember our past, strengthen our relationships, or plan for the future (Kandel, 2006). However, some biased networks contribute to disruption of physiological self-regulation and the limiting of interpretations, choices, actions, and meanings that become possible when considering our past, present, and future.

Interpretation = Perception-Action-Expectation

Perception/action theory (also known as *common-coding theory*) suggests that the processes of perception, action, and expectation share the same interpretative pathways throughout the brain (Proffitt, 2006; Witt, 2011). Networks involved in "receiving" a perception, "doing" a behavior, or "expecting an outcome" all share multidirectional feedback loops that sustain ongoing interpretation focused primarily on the potential outcomes for an individual acting on their surrounding environment.

Affordances (Gibson, 1977) are cognitively coded possibilities for interaction that biased neural networks implicitly construct with an individual's surroundings, providing opportunities for a particular perception or behavior (Chemero, 2003; von Uexküll, 1909). Conversely, expectations about what is possible at any given moment *limit* the range of perceptions, actions, and meanings available to individuals in response to the circumstances of their lives. If "possibilities for action" influence what perceptions/actions might be constructed in the therapeutic process, then scaffolding conversations that attend to narratives similarly "scaffold" neural associations that increase a person's available range of experiences. This helps disrupt familiar, reactive patterns and taken-for-granted perception/action/expectation cycles that diminish both the experience of agency and physiological self-regulation.

Literature from neuroscience has substantiated the role that narratives play in influencing physiology (Barraza, Alexander, Beavin, Terris, & Zak, 2015). Neural networks underlie the perceptual constructs that shape our experience, and we have agency to modify these constructions to support health and wellbeing (Cozolino, 2010). The person becomes an architect of experience rather than a passive receptacle of the world's stimuli.

Narrative Interpretations: The Organizing of Experience

Everything we know and come to know in life is interpreted, and these interpretations shape our lived experience. This is the "narratory principle": humans think, perceive, imagine, and make moral choices according to narrative structures (Sarbin, 1986, p. 8). Narrative therapy (White, 2007; White & Epston, 1990) assumes that we are always engaged in acts of interpretation with others. Our interpretations construct realities through shared schemas of language (Maturana & Varela, 1987) and the constraints of physiology. Persons inhabit the experience of life through narrative meaning; we create "stories" with others that give meaning to our existence.

Narrative interpretations constitute the physiological, interpretive processes of organizing our perceptions, and thereby shape our lived experience and range of available actions. Michael White suggested that our experience is so rich that one story could not express it. Additionally, we suggest narrative interpretations depend on our physiological state. While we may be accustomed to phrases such as "that's the story of my life" (which implies a singular, static understanding of events), one's experience is physically constituted by many ever-shifting stories and physiological states.

Narrative Interpretations and Neuroscience

Interpretation is a physical act that immediately affects our neurophysiology. Every moment we are bombarded with possibilities for living, and most of these go unattended. Only what we find salient and meaningful is included into the neurophysiological process of experiencing life. A primary function of the brain is to selectively ignore most of its surroundings. A large part of brain metabolism is devoted to inhibition (Dorrn, Yuan, Barker, Schreiner, & Froemke, 2010; Salinas & Sejnowski, 2001). If our nervous system did not ignore most available sensory stimuli, we would be overwhelmed and unable to function.

Over time, physiologies are established that correspond to familiar narrative interpretations about ourselves, the trajectory of our lives, relationships, health, our ability to regulate our bodies, and our sense of agency. When perceptual networks that participate in language, memory, sensory perception, and affect become integrated, we are able to tell a meaningful narrative (Cozolino, 2010). This highlights the physiology of narrative interpretations. Our lived experience interacts with the diverse sensory and cognitive aspects of our lives, creating a coherent set of associations that guide our actions and expectations for the future.

Narrative Neurotherapy: Scaffolding, Learning, and Neurophysiology

White (2007) describes scaffolding in terms of movement or transport from one place to another (see also Duvall & Béres, 2011). Rather than a flash of insight, he offers the *migration of identity* metaphor—a journey from one location in time to another, and from one experience of identity to another. The outcome is an increasing range of available behaviors towards certain preferred identities, actions, and experiences. White maintains that the *Zone of Proximal Development* can be crossed by way of conversational partnerships, which support persons distancing themselves from their immediate experience of problems. When persons are not caught up in the vortex of immediate experience, they are positioned to use their skills of meaning making to direct their lives according to what they place value upon. "It is this conceptual development that supplies the foundation for people to regulate their lives: to influence their own actions in purposeful ways, to intervene in their own lives to shape the course of events, and to problem-solve" (White, 2007, p. 272). While White refers to the conceptual processes necessary to regulate our lives, we are emphasizing the neurophysiological processes necessary for this to occur. This suggests attention to the *landscape of physiology*, as well as the *landscapes of action and identity* traditionally referenced by narrative therapists.

Movements of Narrative Neurotherapy: Scaffolding Identity States

NNT scaffolding conversations promote separating from problem-identity states in order to develop alternative identity states. We are suggesting three movements that spiral forward and loop back rather than a linear progression. A brief description of recent work between myself (Jan) and Tom will illustrate the practices of Narrative Neurotherapy. This was a year-long transition (20 sessions) toward sustained change in Tom's physiology and identity. Tom moved from anxious, depressed identity states of "Failure" (including persistent stomach problems) to inhabiting an identity state of "Calm Confidence" with clarity of his life initiatives and a resolution of physiological symptoms.

Movement 1: Separating from Immediate Problem-Identity States

Practices

Make distinctions about physical sensations. Associate distinctions with identity states. Contextualize to connect sociocultural discourses with physiology. Separate from the physiology of urgency. Invite settled, reflective physiology. Notice and name preferred identity states. Support preferred identity states and stalled initiatives. Consider community.

MAKE DISTINCTIONS ABOUT PHYSICAL SENSATIONS

Tom is a 47-year-old white male who stated he was "depressed . . . I might need to take a drastic step of trying medication." I listened for expressions regarding his physiology. Cultural and professional discourses promote binary thinking about mind versus body, encouraging therapists to ignore or feel powerless to impact physiological symptoms. Tom's stomach problems interrupted daily living. He inquired about a prescription but considered pharmaceuticals a "last resort." His primary physician regarded this as "probably stress related" and "psychological." I asked Tom if we could settle into conversations, paying attention to his physiology.

ASSOCIATE DISTINCTIONS WITH IDENTITY STATES

Tom explained he had left a "stressful job" as a CEO, "noticing feeling down and panicky" along "with stomach problems." During his workday he would "start to feel really down and negative about life and would want to go home and go to bed." Months after his job ended, symptoms persisted. Tom stated, "I have a constant knot in my stomach. . . . I took a big hit last year with a job failure." Job loss and stomach problems were interwoven. Stress, anxiety, muscle tension, fatigue, upset stomach, low self esteem, negative thinking were all effects of this profound "hit." I asked what conclusions he was coming to about himself regarding this series of events. Tom stated:

> "Great CEOs turn businesses around. I couldn't do that. . . . I pretty much feel like a failure of a man. . . . I have a fear of failure now. . . .

I've lost confidence in myself. . . . (I) can't take action necessary to create a new job. . . . nothing I do makes a difference."

The interpretations and accompanying physiology of failure dominated how he was experiencing himself and his situation. We noticed an identity of "Failure" had distinct sensations and physiology, constraining Tom's ability to make changes he would prefer.

CONTEXTUALIZE TO CONNECT SOCIOCULTURAL DISCOURSES
WITH PHYSIOLOGY

Often I ask myself, *how might we think about this?* Reflective conversations require a distinct physical state, interrupting the conclusive and often panicked physiology of immediate problem-solving. Positioning problems within sociocultural contexts can shift physiology, loosen dominant problem stories, and generate material for new narrative interpretations. I wondered how "success" and "failure" were being understood in his roles as a businessman and husband in a heterosexual marriage. Culturally defined gender roles can be both expanding and limiting to identities (Ewing & Allen, 2009). *Managing* money, *controlling* finances, *making* decisions, and *functioning* independently were actions associated with Tom's constructions of a "successful" identity. We situated his job loss in a larger context. How was loss of employment stressful and disorienting as a male provider? Who was supporting him? At first, these contextual questions seemed startling and unfamiliar to Tom.

SUPPORTING PREFERRED IDENTITY STATES AND STALLED INITIATIVES

When telling and re-telling problem stories, stalled initiatives are less visible but nonetheless present. These initiatives have become dormant due to circumstances and physiological states that initially appear outside of one's control. Early on Tom stated, "I'm not sure if I kind of left or was fired." These two interpretations could produce different meanings and identity states. If he had left because he was unhappy, then his corresponding physiological state seemed more energetic and hopeful. If he was fired, he felt immobile and "sick." I asked Tom about wanting to leave his job and he said he "didn't like it," "felt evaluated," and had to "sacrifice a lot to be in my position." Why was the stalled initiative of "wanting to leave" not getting attention?

A Therapist Might Consider

Persons talking in ways that seem conclusive of their identities and constraining of their ability to take action. Problem-saturated urgent language, problematic sensations/physiology. Limited narratives of possible actions.

Physical expressions ranging from panic, fatigue, or rapid speech, to settled, clear, energized. Contrasting preferred and problem physiologies.

Applicable Neuroscience

Nervous systems reorganize with new experiences. Enriched environments (Garthe, Roeder, & Kempermann, 2015) facilitate growth of neurophysiological connections and create a stimulus for new learning and identity states. States of urgency often disregulate physiology and make reflection about complex concepts difficult: a link exists between the sympathetic nervous system and inhibition of frontal cortex involvement in problem-solving (Arnsten, 2009; Hänsel & Känel, 2008).

Movement 2: Substantiating Intentional Identity States

Practices

Name and thicken interpretations that further substantiate preferred identity states. Associate and evaluate any physiological sensations that are related to new interpretations or actions. Recognize and thicken stalled initiatives and associated states. Identify actions supporting preferred identity states. Notice developing practices that support preferred changes. Loop back to Movement 1 if problem-identity states resurface.

NAME AND THICKEN INTERPRETATIONS THAT FURTHER
SUBSTANTIATE PREFERRED IDENTITY STATES

By session 4, Tom had begun noticing sociocultural effects that allowed for new interpretations, stating:

> "I'm becoming more comfortable with what happened in my CEO role and I don't want it to define me. . . . I don't need to think of it that way. . . . I've become more comfortable admitting the environmental influence."

Tom associated dominant sociocultural notions of being a *businessman* and *provider* with feeling "uptight":

> "I felt demands to be independent as a business leader . . . to put work first . . . [to] always know what I was doing. . . . [to] not feel like I should ask for help. . . . [to] have it together."

He referred to considering these sociocultural influences as Expanded Thinking. He mentioned "feeling better," a little lighter and less depressed, whenever he could access Expanded Thinking.

ASSOCIATE AND EVALUATE ANY PHYSIOLOGICAL SENSATIONS THAT
ARE RELATED TO NEW INTERPRETATIONS OR ACTIONS

Why was it helpful for Tom to consider Expanded Thinking? He said, "This new perspective gives me confidence. . . . allows me to be more optimistic about myself. . . . helps me not feel like I'm not smart, or an underachiever, or can't meet challenges."

J: Tell me more about this idea of confidence? Can you describe it?
T: It's a calmness in my body. I'm thinking clearly. I'm slower; it means I can figure it out and find solutions to things. I can change some of the weakness of myself. I can believe in my abilities. I can be more patient with myself and others. I'm not criticizing myself so harshly; it's not being egotistical, self absorbed, but it's being with a peaceful assurance of your ability to tackle the task or circumstances.
J: So you are referring to this moment when there is a calmness and you know you have the ability to tackle things or problem-solve as confidence?
T: It's kind of a calm confidence.

Tom names and experiences a preference for Calm Confidence, both as a physical state and an interpretation of his identity. We discussed experiences of Calm Confidence as it appears throughout his job search and his relationship to wife and children, noticing that Expanded Thinking supports Calm Confidence.

Calm Confidence helped Tom initiate numerous actions: finding an employment headhunter, actively searching for job leads, exploring job opportunities, and interviewing with several companies. Subsequent conversations focused on specific job interviews, where I invited him to evaluate what sensations fit for him and what opportunities felt right to pursue. I gave close attention to these actions, asking him to name the effects on his life and his physiology. Throughout this process, Tom noted "take-aways" indicating he was learning something important about his preference for Calm Confidence and the possibilities it created.

A Therapist Might Consider

Persons more fully associating physiology with their actions and identities. Persons mentioning additional realizations, learnings, knowings about their sensed experience. Referencing sensations when speaking of what they are doing and who is surrounding them.

Applicable Neuroscience

New neural connections are strengthened through repetition over extended periods of time. Regulated physiological states lead to more reflective interpretations of experience (Grawe, 2007). Neural associations between preferred physiological sensations and states of identity can be created and strengthened. Repeated new experiences will disrupt biased perception/action loops built into problem-saturated stories, allowing new possibilities for action.

Movement 3: Inhabiting Preferred Identity States

Practices

Notice physiological differences between past and present identity states. Loop back to previous movements to fortify new identity states. Revisit named intentions. Notice developing daily habits that support preferred identity states. Hypothesize/imagine future possibilities. Include community. Consider resources needed to sustain changes. Invite predictions about what could now be possible.

NOTICING PHYSIOLOGICAL DIFFERENCES BETWEEN
PAST AND PRESENT IDENTITY STATES

I asked Tom, "So you have been noticing some ways that you have sustained more Calm Confidence? And you wanted to recognize that's a change for you?" He replied:

> "[I'm] just working on Calm Confidence again and again . . . in the beginning I was sometimes feeling like I'm really doing a crappy job. But I feel I've got a number of examples now where I'm really staying a lot more calm and even when I'm having periods of stress I'm recognizing it. And you know, that's really critical. . . . You have helped me to think about those things differently . . . I've now done this 80 times so shouldn't I been getting a little better at it? I know that Calm Confidence is something we can learn how to do effectively."

LOOP BACK TO PREVIOUS MOVEMENTS TO FORTIFY NEW IDENTITY STATES

One of Tom's job interviews advances to the point of negotiating a salary and expecting a formal offer. When the job offer dissolved, he consulted with me about feeling badly and the reappearance of "Failure to Succeed" saying "I started feeling down and anxious." Although Tom began telling his story of Failure, he also spoke of his apprehensions. Why didn't he just take the job at a reduced salary? Why didn't the job seem to fit with what he preferred?

J: I want to understand more about the job position. As you were negotiating the job, it became clear that things were not feeling right, that things weren't quite adding up?

T: Yeah, the salary wasn't within range, the communication between the CEO and headhunter became unclear, they didn't really have a great accounting system, they didn't really have many committed people, they asked me to oversee manufacturing and operations, I'd be traveling a lot in the beginning. So there was some part like oh man, this is a lot! But I told myself but Tom you can do it.

J: So you were willing to try to make it work even though it wasn't feeling right, it wasn't quite adding up to what you had in mind? And you had concerns?

T: Yes, this was an opportunity, but do I really want to go back into all of this?

J: You had said earlier that you wanted something different, so do you really want to go back into this kind of situation?

T: Yeah but I couldn't think that then. That was hard to ask.

I reminded Tom of his previous statements of preference when he was reflecting on his next work situation. He said, "Life is too short to do this type of work. I sacrificed a lot." He had wanted more flexibility and to know that his work made a difference. Revisiting this, Tom said, "Yeah, where I sit right now I see it that way and I'm not that upset. I see [it] clearer now that we are discussing it."

HYPOTHESIZE, IMAGINE FUTURE POSSIBILITIES

Before his second-to-last session, Tom accepted a job offer, and his new schedule made it difficult to continue sessions. I invited Tom to speak of the future in relation to his experiences of Calm Confidence.

T: I'd say today is a day of awareness. We are reviewing the past year and reviewing where we are with Calm Confidence. How do we continue to encourage it or the indirect encouragement? And the amazing thing is I actually feel really good right now.

J: Okay, so maybe we continue to discuss how Calm Confidence is present, and how it continues to be present and noticing how are you doing that. I imagine it's a part of your life most of the time now. It's getting implemented in different ways. If you imagine Calm Confidence to continue on in your life through the years, what do you think could come of that? How might your life be different?

T: Well, I think it would make me a better father, a better husband, a better overall person, a better leader. In every facet of my life this would be true. I'd feel better too.

J: Does anyone else know that you have claimed this piece of identity that you are wanting to stay close to? That you are wanting to become part of you more and more? Do you think your wife is picking up on these changes?

T: Well I have mentioned it to her. I mean I have all of this all over my closet. I have the goals we have outlined in here, and I have Calm Confidence right in the middle. I have like six sheets on my wall in my closet. . . . I want to give myself a lot of credit because it has been a beast for a long time. It's good when you start down a path and it starts to germinate within you and you start to have some success, and then you feel good about that, and the way you are interacting makes you feel good and that combination of having some success keeps you going. And you can say "I like that!" I think that's a better me! I like what that feels like. I like what that looks like, I like how that interacts with others, and how it lifts up other people. Feeling like I am making a lot of progress there and therefore that has been really buoying my spirit up a lot to feel like I'm having a lot of success there. I can tell that my mood's better, I can tell that as I even start to think about some stressful elements I'm not letting my mind go into the deep holes of irrationality as much. But I feel like my temperament and my Calm Confidence is better, like with my reactions. You know the sky isn't falling as much. And that I attribute more to our conversations and me thinking things through better. Calm Confidence! Well, Jan, let me fill you in (laughing), that there are a lot of ways to look at certain events and one certain event shouldn't be your whole definition of who you are. So if you will broaden your perspective a little bit, you might have some recognition that perhaps even within some failure there were some great benefits.

J: So there's another story? (laughing) How's your stomach been?

T: It's been really good. It hasn't been a problem.

A Therapist Might Consider

Persons feeling more confident, settled, physiologically regulated. Incorporating previous intentions into their habits and practices of daily living. Expressing possibilities for taking action. Making predictions about their future in ways that acknowledge their own agency. Collecting resources (e.g., formulating specific plans, finding allies) to support new initiatives.

Applicable Neuroscience

Repetition is critical. Developing practices and habits, combined with the experience of inhabiting new identity states, correspond to the strengthening of new neural networks. Development of inhibiting brain connections between the prefrontal cortex and learned reactions of the nervous system (Gass & Chandler, 2013), resulting in increased self-regulation and implicit habits of well-regulated physiology.

Conclusion

Scaffolding identity states is the intentional act of bringing potentialities of narrative material into a storyline while recognizing physiological, relational, cultural, and environmental contexts. Narrative Neurotherapy is situated between social constructionist and scientific theories, with an emphasis on physiology and learning rather than healing. Neurophysiological research indicates that all perception is interpretive and intricately involved with the narrative organization that shapes identity states. NNT scaffolding conversations promote narrative interpretations that align with what persons place value upon and correspond with preferred states of identity. These narrative interpretations support repeated preferred actions, making a neurophysiological context that sustains preferred changes over time. Neuron by neuron, we are able to inhabit a new experience of life through the infinite connections we share with the world.

References

Arnsten, A. F. (2009). Stress signalling pathways that impair prefrontal cortex structure and function. *Nature Reviews Neuroscience, 10*(6), 410–422.

Bailey, C. H., Bartsch, D., & Kandel, E. R. (1996). Toward a molecular definition of long-term memory storage. *Proceedings of the National Academy of Sciences, 39*(24), 13445–13452.

Barraza, J., Alexander, V., Beavin, L., Terris, E., & Zak, P. (2015). The heart of the story: Peripheral physiology during narrative exposure predicts charitable giving. *Biological Psychology, 105,* 138–143.

Chemero, A. (2003). An outline of a theory of affordances. *Ecological Psychology, 15*(2), 181–195.

Cozolino, L. (2010). *The neuroscience of psychotherapy: Healing the social brain* (2nd ed.). New York, NY: W. W. Norton & Company Inc.

Dorrn, A. L., Yuan, K., Barker, A. J., Schreiner, C. E., & Froemke, R. C. (2010). Developmental sensory experience balances cortical excitation and inhibition. *Nature, 465,* 932–936.

Duvall, J., & Béres, L. (2011). Storied therapy as a three-act play. In *Innovations in narrative therapy: Connecting practice, training, and research* (pp. 37–90). New York, NY: W. W. Norton & Company Inc.

Ewing, J., & Allen, K. (2009). Women's narratives about god and gender: Agency, tension, and change. *Journal of Systemic Therapies, 27*(3), 95–112.

Garthe, A., Roeder, I., & Kempermann, G. (2015). Mice in an enriched environment learn more flexibly because of adult hippocampal neurogenesis. *Hippocampus, 26*(2), 261–271.

Gass, J. T., & Chandler, L. J. (2013). The plasticity of extinction: Contribution of the prefrontal cortex in treating addiction through inhibitory learning. *Front Psychiatry, 4*(46), 1–13.

Gibson, J. J. (1977). The theory of affordances. In R. Shaw & J. Bransford (Eds.), *Perceiving, acting, and knowing* (pp. 127–135). Hillsdale, NJ: Lawrence Erlbaum Associates Publishers.

Gluck, M., Mercado, E., & Myers, C. (2008). The neuroscience of learning and memory. In *Learning and memory: From brain to behavior* (pp. 44–77). New York, NY: Worth Publishers.

Grawe, K. (2007). *Neuropsychotherapy: How the neurosciences inform effective psychotherapy*. Mahwah, NJ: Lawrence Erlbaum Associates Publishers.

Hänsel, A., & Känel, R. (2008). The ventro-medial prefrontal cortex: A major link between the autonomic nervous system, regulation of emotion, and stress reactivity? *BioPsychoSocial Medicine, 2*(1), 21.

Hebb, D. (1949). *The organization of behavior: A neuropsychological theory.* New York, NY: John Wiley & Sons.

Kandel, E. (2006). *In search of memory: The emergence of a new science of mind.* New York, NY: W. W. Norton & Company Inc.

Kozorovitskiy, Y., Gross, C. G., & Kopil, C. (2005). Experience induces structural and biochemical changes in the adult primate brain. *Proceedings of the National Academy of Sciences, 102*(48), 17478–17482.

LeDoux, J. E. (2002). *Synaptic self: How our brains become who we are.* New York, NY: Viking.

Maturana, H. R., & Varela, F. J. (1987). *The tree of knowledge: The biological roots of human understanding.* Boston, MA: Shambhala Publications.

Paulsen, O., & Sejnowski, T. J. (2000). Natural patterns of activity and long-term synaptic plasticity. *Current Opinion in Neurobiology, 10*(2), 172–179.

Proffitt, D. (2006). Embodied perception and the economy of action. *Perspectives on Psychological Science, 1*(2), 110–122.

Salinas, E., & Sejnowski, T. J. (2001). Correlated neuronal activity and the flow of neural information. *National Review of Neuroscience, 22,* 539–550.

Sarbin, T. (1986). *Narrative psychology the storied nature of human conduct.* New York, NY: Praeger Publishers/Greenwood Publishing Group.

von Uexküll, J. (1909). Umwelt und Innenwelt der Tiere. [trans. Environment and the inner world of animals]. Berlin: Springer-Verlag.

Vygotsky, L. (1962). *Thought and language.* Cambridge, MA: MIT Press.

Vygotsky, L. (1978). Interaction between learning and development. In E. Souberman, S. Scribner, & V. John-Steiner (Eds.), *Mind and society* (pp. 79–91). Cambridge, MA: Harvard University Press.

White, M. (2007). *Maps of narrative practice.* New York, NY: W. W. Norton & Company Inc.

White, M., & Epston, D. (1990). *Narrative means to therapeutic ends.* New York, NY: W. W. Norton & Company Inc.

Witt, J. K. (2011). Action's effect on perception. *Current Directions in Psychological Science, 20*(3), 201–206.

Wood, D., Bruner, J. S., & Ross, G. (1976). The role of tutoring in problem solving. *Journal of Child Psychology and Psychiatry, 17,* 89–100.

Section II

Research, Questions, and Theoretical Dilemmas Which can Inform Clinical Practices

8 Single Session Therapy and Neuroscience

Scaffolding and Social Engagement

Karen Young, Jim Hibel, Jaime Tartar, and Mercedes Fernandez

Introduction

Brief narrative practices are becoming one of the most utilized collaborative approaches in walk-in therapy clinics and single session therapy across Ontario, Canada (Duvall & Young, 2015; Duvall, Young, & Kayes-Burden, 2012; Young, 2011b). The deliberate attention to scaffolding questions that create movement toward new understandings is a cornerstone of narrative practice (White, 2007) and one that is key in providing meaningful change in single session counseling (Young, 2008, 2011a). These scaffolded brief conversations establish a partnership between the client and therapist as the therapist proposes incremental questions that co-create new knowledge. The process is highly collaborative, relational, and social, all necessary components for meaningful outcomes in brief therapy (Duvall & Young, 2015; Hubble, Duncan, & Miller, 1999; Lambert, Shapiro, & Bergin, 1994; Orlinsky, Grawe, & Parks, 1994). Recent literature has been illuminating important intersections between the growing knowledge in neuroscience and both well-established and innovative practices in narrative therapy (Beaudoin & Zimmerman, 2011; Cozolino, 2010; Maclennan, 2015; Zimmerman & Beaudoin, 2015).

The brain, its anatomy and processes, and their relationships to consciousness and behavior have been studied for over a century (Cozolino, 2010). Narrative therapy has also been written about since its emergence in the early 1980s (White, 1989, 2007). These disciplines have remained on parallel paths, occupying separate epistemological territories. The recent work of Daniel Siegel and his contemporaries have brought forward findings that have the potential to cross the boundaries of these epistemological territories; a process that Siegel refers to as "consilience"—the bringing together of areas of interest that have previously been separate (2012).

In new research in the area of neuroscience and single session therapy, we are discovering evidence that supports powerful neuro-biological effects of brief narrative conversations. The use of narrative practice maps offers clients a good workout, "stretch[ing] his or her mind" (White, 2007, p. 272), and facilitates strong social engagement. This social engagement is created through a focused attention on novel conversations that includes new ways to perceive problems and strengthens connections to cherished values and commitments. This "enriched environment" (Cozolino, 2010, p. 20) results in optimal conditions for change. Our research demonstrates the neuro-biological effects of such an enriched therapeutic environment within single session therapy.

In this chapter we describe the practice of scaffolding in narrative therapy and its importance in creating social engagement in single session therapy. We demonstrate through past research that scaffolding is present in single session therapy and outline the therapeutic effects of this for brief therapy. Then we explore the neuro-biological effects of scaffolding on social engagement and elaborate this as shown through new research that looked at the effects of this kind of conversation on EEG measures and changes in alpha-amylase and cortisol. We close with some exploration of the impacts of the research findings on our clinical work and on our teaching.

The Importance of Scaffolding and Social Engagement in Single Sessions

In single session work at walk-in clinics or in other brief service delivery contexts (Duvall, Young, & Kayes-Burden, 2012), we have an obligation to those consulting us to do more than just gather information and assess, as in many more traditional initial contacts. We have a responsibility to create an impactful, meaningful, and useful therapeutic encounter within the single contact. This is a complex task that requires therapists to position themselves collaboratively and with a competency-oriented curiosity, to co-develop a purpose or agenda for the conversation, and then to embark on a journey that moves everyone present toward new understandings and experience (Duvall & Young, 2015; Young, 2011a). This movement or journey within a brief narrative single session is supported though scaffolding conversations.

In his later writings, Michael White (2006, 2007) made extensive reference to the work of Russian psychologist Lev Vygotsky (1978, 1987). Indeed, the increasing use of ideas and terms such as distancing, space, scaffolding, and social collaboration in his work reflected a Vygotskian re-visioning of his conversations maps (Ramey, Young, & Tarulli, 2010). Vygotsky (1978) emphasized that learning was an achievement not of independent effort but of social collaboration. The gap between what is currently known and what is possible to know is traversed within relationships—within social collaboration with another person who guides or scaffolds the person across the gap.

Scaffolding conversations are organized according to a map with a hierarchy beginning with naming and characterizing the problem or initiative, referred to as "low-level distancing" (White, 2006, p. 45). This marks the early stages of concept formation, as unthematized and unconnected experiences are united under a common name or category (Ramey et al., 2010). The name and description of both problems and initiatives invited forward in these conversations are both novel and experience-near. Clients experience novelty as the therapist asks questions in ways that separate persons from the problems, externalizing problems. Externalized problem descriptions are experience-near as the person develops their own new language, often including metaphor and images. Initiatives are described in detail, finding new language that is moving, meaningful, and, again, experience-near. This high degree of novelty and emotionally experience-near unique problem and initiatives talk is highly engaging (Beaudoin & Zimmerman, 2011; White, 2007; Young, 2008).

In this example of a session with a 15-year-old female, "Jane" and myself (KY), we can see the presence of scaffolded questions. We first explore questions that name and describe. Initially in response to questions about the problem, she described "the problem with not eating," moving to "the low self esteem" and then to "the self criticism."

K: Jane, when you think about all of this (her words on a page), what do you think you might call this problem if it had an overarching name?

J: (Pausing and thinking) Well, I think it should probably be called "Anorexia."

K: If you could describe it, like an image or picture, what would Anorexia look like?

J: It would be a dark, kinda foggy thing . . . it's hard to see it, it looks like it is smiling, but it also looks a little mean and sneaky. And it sits on my shoulder all the time.

Medium-level distancing is the next step in the map, and these tasks produce chains of association between the problem or initiative and its consequences, as the effects of the problem or initiative are explored (Ramey et al., 2010). The effects are explored in detail and again new and novel understandings about the problem, self, and relationships emerge.

K: What would Anorexia want for your life if it could get you in its grip?

J: I don't know . . . (thoughtful)

K: Would Anorexia want you to feel good about eating?

J: No.

K: Would Anorexia want you to feel good about yourself inside?

J: No.

K: How would Anorexia want you to feel?

J: Probably worse, bad about myself, so I got worse. . . . I was just feed-
ing it. I guess . . . the more I don't eat the more it feeds!

K: Ya. So the way you feed Anorexia is by feeling worse and worse
about yourself, that's what it likes? (Nods.) What do you think it
ultimately wants for your life?

J: (Long pause, thoughtful) Probably death.

Medium-high-level distancing tasks then invite the person to evaluate the effects of the problem or initiative. Then in high-level distancing tasks, clients are invited to justify and explain their evaluations. At
both these levels, connections are made to preferences, values, commitments, and relationships with others. These conversations that touch
on what matters to people, what they stand for, relationships that have
been significant and inspiring in their life and so on are highly emotionally charged and moving. When we facilitate this within single session therapy, we have created a space for significant and meaningful
realizations that can make a difference in people's lives. Very high-level
distancing tasks then invite clients to make plans of action based on
the newly understood concepts, realizations, and the preferences for
their lives that they are now in touch with (Duvall & Young, 2009;
White, 2007).

K: Is that different from what you want for your life, Jane?

J: Yes.

K: Can you describe for me the different life you want?

Jane describes a life full of friendship, family, laughter, travel, a job she
enjoys, and feeling good about herself. She calls it a "good life."

K: This "good" life you have described, would it include room for an
Anorexic sort of lifestyle in any way?

J: No, no way. It would take away the good life.

Later in the conversation I introduce questions that explore values.

K: Are there some ideas that society has that have kind of fed Anorexia's
critical thoughts?

J: Ya. A lot of people in today's society only look at your appearance,
like how your body looks. So a lot of it has to do with other people's
judgment.

K: Do you think that society tries to dictate to people about how they
should look?

J: Ya, for sure.

K: What do you think our society dictates to women about how they
should look?

J: A lot of it is about the make-up and clothing, and having good bodies that are perfect. Like on T.V., and if you don't look like that then
you're nobody. (pauses, thinking)

K: What do you think about these expectations—are they reasonable,
unreasonable?

J: I think they're unreasonable, cause not everyone can have a perfect
body, or a perfect face, and it's just wrong, because if it's not possible
for them then they feel they can't be anybody. It's just not right.

K: Can you say some more about why you see this as so unreasonable,
and not right?

J: Well, because that's what happened to me, cause I just got dragged
into it, into the thoughts to want to be like that. There is so much
stuff going on about how you look, not how you are inside, that's
really bad—you shouldn't be judged on how you look—well actually, you shouldn't really be judged at all, so . . . (pauses). I think
now I can see myself getting over it. The voices that say, "Don't' eat,
hate yourself, starve," they're still there, but they're not voicing their
opinion as loudly, like, a whisper, before they were yelling going Jane
you're fat, don't eat at all, starve yourself . . . now they are just talking, but quieter.

The movement within the scaffolding map is fluid, from naming and
description to effects, possibly returning to naming again, and then to
evaluation of effects and the reasons or justification for the evaluation.
The flexible and creative use of scaffolding in single session therapy is
highly socially engaging, supporting the client to see problems with new
eyes, to connect their responses and initiatives to their values and preferences, and to envision ways to move forward in ways that are in keeping
with these preferences.

Research on the Presence of Scaffolding
in Single Sessions

The presence of scaffolding in brief narrative single session therapy is not
only a claim but has been substantiated by research. In 2010 White's scaffolding conversations map inspired the following research questions: Do
narrative therapy sessions demonstrate the type of conversation described
in White's scaffolding conversations map? If so, do children respond to
therapists' scaffolding by responding to therapists' questions at the same
level of the map? Finally, do therapists and children proceed through the
steps of the map over the course of a single session (Ramey et al., 2010)?
Observational coding was used to test White's scaffolding conversations
map against actual process in single sessions of therapy with children.
The findings showed that most speech turns were codable at some level
of the map, that children responded to therapists' scaffolding, and that

therapists and children tended to proceed through the steps of the map in single session therapy. These findings demonstrated that White's model of therapy is observable and suggested that change occurred at the level of language over the session. This established the presence of scaffolding as a consistent practice in brief narrative single sessions.

Neuro-Biological Effects of Scaffolding on Social Engagement

In single session work, the use of scaffolding assists therapists to create a conversation that has immediate and sufficient movement into new knowledge, concepts, and experience, thereby increasing the likelihood of the single conversation being highly engaging and therefore impactful and useful. The pace in these single sessions is deliberately slow, to allow for sufficient rich description and realizations to emerge through a type of guided "loitering" (White, p. 234) in meaningful conversation.

There are any number of internal experiences that take place during this loitering that have been linked to neurophysiological factors; for example: attention, novelty, relevance and repetition (Beaudoin, 2010); emotional/affective engagement (Beaudoin & Zimmerman, 2011); mindfulness and regulation (Hanson & Mendius, 2009); and implicit memories and receptivity (Badenoch, 2011). It is likely that inviting a new or novel name and a rich, detailed description that closely reflects the person's affective and cognitive experience results in more immediately impactful and sustained effects of the therapeutic conversation. Naming an experience is associated with a reduction of amygdala activity and the brain's increased ability to regulate (Beaudoin & Zimmerman, 2011). What White refers to as an "experience-near" (2007, p. 40) or "rich characterization" (Duvall & Young, 2009, p. 7) regarding the naming and description of problems and initiatives is important within single sessions. Research has found that novelty triggers curiosity and a release of dopamine in the brain, a neurotransmitter associated with positive experiences (Beaudoin, 2010). Discoveries in neuroscience strongly support the effects of rich, experience-near descriptions. Siegel writes:

> We . . . [use] words to access the wordless right hemisphere realm of sensations, images, and feelings. . . . When we *explain* a science experiment . . . we are relying heavily on the left [hemisphere]. When we *describe* rather than explain, we are bringing the experientially rich right side into collaboration with the word-smithing left hemisphere.
> (2011, p. 114)

This linking of words, affect, images, and sensations is key, as it links "left and right, not replac[ing] one imbalance with another" (p. 116) but bringing the hemispheres into relationship, which supports optimal functioning (Siegel & Bryson, 2012). These experience-near descriptions developed in single sessions are usually both externalized problem descriptions and as well new powerful words and language for initiatives and responses people have engaged in. This introduces novelty, which Siegel suggests is important:

> Novelty, or exposing ourselves to new ideas and experiences, promotes the growth of new connections among existing neurons and seems to stimulate the growth of myelin, the fatty sheath that speeds nerve transmissions. Novelty can even stimulate the growth of new neurons.
>
> (2011, p. 84)

The deliberately slow, experience-near (perhaps this could be described as emotionally near) novel language development, and the at times repetitive movement up and down in scaffolded conversations, creates the conditions for neuroplasticity, the ability of the brain to change its structure in response to experience (Siegel, 2011; Siegel, 2012). We are facilitating focused attention, repetition, novelty, and emotional arousal—all essential for learning, concept development, and neuroplasticity (Beaudoin & Zimmerman, 2011; Siegel, 2011). Cozolino (2010) writes that enthusiasm and curiosity are the best states for learning. As we ask interesting questions within a supported context, we create an "optimal arousal" (p. 46) in the form of curiosity and enthusiasm and "these motivated states have all been recognized for their role in successful outcomes in psychotherapy" (p. 46). Narratives are collaboratively co-constructed, building and re-building neural structures, such that Cozolino proposes psychotherapy as a neurobiological intervention (p. 305). We would venture that these effects of curiosity, enthusiasm, collaboration, and optimal arousal could also be described as a high degree of social engagement, a condition that we would propose as essential for impactful therapeutic encounters in single sessions.

Research on the Neuro-Biological Effects of Scaffolding

In this spirit of consilience between brief narrative practices and neuroscience, we have considered the ways in which the kinds of conversations that take place within narrative single sessions might be observable from a neuroscience perspective. It has been demonstrated that single sessions can be observed to engage participants along the lines of the scaffolding map (Ramey et al., 2010). We were interested in research that might demonstrate that conversations that included elements of scaffolding conversations have observable and measurable neurophysiological effects.

Siegel (2011, 2012) considers relationship to be one of the cornerstones of mind. This notion of the relational brain is one of the points of intersection that has caught the interest of narrative therapists. The various maps of narrative practice, including the scaffolding map, as described above, collaboratively engage people in unique, novel, and meaningful conversations. These kinds of questions and engagement fit well with Siegel's and Cozolino's notions of engagement and creating a space that encourages enhancement of neurological functioning. Physiologically, events that are novel and engaging encourage the development of new pathways in the brain. New pathways of interconnected neurons are literally created within the brain in response to environmental stimulation as well as the development of new synapses and brain cells themselves (Cozolino, 2010; Siegel, 2012). Relational involvement and social engagement seem to be at the heart of these processes, and at the heart of single session therapy, as we need to make the most of the session by creating a high degree of social engagement immediately.

A Biological Measure of Social Engagement

There has been a recent groundswell of support for the observation that the processes described by Siegel and others fit smoothly with the intentions and practices of narrative therapy (Zimmerman & Beaudoin, 2015), and that these areas of overlap can be readily and richly described. Along with these observations, we became interested in seeing if elements of these conversations could be observed to have the sorts of neurophysiological effects that we expected might take place within single sessions of brief narrative therapy. In particular, we sought to identify some neurophysiological markers that would be consistent with the kinds of social and relational engagement that we would expect to arise in scaffolding conversations. For this purpose, we chose to look at two biological markers and one assessment of brain activity.

One of the two biological markers we assayed was salivary cortisol, a chemical that is elevated under periods of social arousal, and which has been implicated in adverse effects over long periods of stress. We also assayed levels of salivary alpha-amylase, a more rapidly responding marker of social arousal, or "fight or flight," in more intense events. More recently, it has become understood that these markers are also reflective of social engagement, when the person is involved in interesting and meaningful experiences over a more brief period (Hibel, Trumbell, & Mercado, 2014; Shirtcliff, Peres, Dismukes, Lee, & Phan, 2014). We also collected data on EEG patterns, which we analyzed at seven levels of brain activity. There is considerable research on biomarkers such as cortisol and alpha-amylase, as well as on EEG patterns related to different affective and attentional states (Arita, 2012; Howells, Ives-Deliperi, Horn, & Stein, 2012; Lutz et al., 2013; Miskovic et al., 2011; Moscovitch et al., 2011; Sobolewski, Holt, Kublik, & Wróbel, 2011), which support the notions that conversations that take place within a scaffolding context that provide novelty, naming, and other components of social engagement would have measurable effects.

The study took place at Nova Southeastern University, a large private, not-for profit University in Florida, as a collaboration between Jim Hibel (who is a professor in the Marriage and Family Therapy Program) and Drs. Fernandez and Tartar (who are research and teaching neuroscientists in other departments in the university). The study itself took place in a research lab where volunteers attended to engage in a conversation with Jim Hibel, while EEG and salivary samples were taken. We divided participants into two situations. In one situation, the conversations were neutral ("describe campus architecture" or "describe your typical day"). These were intended to be as different as possible from a scaffolding conversation and served as a comparison group. For the second situation, participants each engaged in a single conversation with JH that was guided by narrative scaffolding concepts. These conversations were divided into two parts, and EEG and biomarkers were assessed before and after each part.

The first part of the single conversation was aligned with near-level distancing tasks in which participants were asked incremental questions that explored the question, "Think of a problem, challenge, or difficulty that you have faced in your life that you have had success with, or that you have triumphed over." The questions that were asked were designed to bring forward an experience-near problem description, involving naming the challenge, placing the challenge in time and place, and mapping the effects of the problem on the person. As a pathway towards middle-level distancing, participants were also asked about the aspects of the problem that conflicted with their preferences for life; what made this a problem for them.

The second part of the conversation invoked medium-high-level distancing questions. Here, the focus was on the success or the triumph. These conversations invited the person to evaluate the effects that they had on the problem, including specifics about the triumph, their role in the triumph, and the involvement and responses of important others to their successful initiatives. Additionally, consistent with high-level distancing conversations, the conversations included questions about the participant's preferences, values, commitments, and relationships with others. Below is a brief, edited transcript of one of these conversations.

Evan (name changed for privacy) attended a single session conversation with JH. This session did not take place in a therapy context. Rather, Evan was a participant in the research project, and was not seeking help for any particular problem. However, part of the presuppositions that underlie our collaborative work assumes that there is generally little that distinguishes a "client" from a "normal" person, other than circumstances and intentions in seeking consultations. We do not see persons working on problems as "other." For this reason, it was not surprising that individuals who attended this research project were readily able to bring forward personal, evocative, and often moving stories of their difficulties, as well as their triumphs.

In this case, Evan told of his experience of "refugee isolation and despair," including the effects on his life of fear, disconnection from his familiar home and from his family, and many practical life challenges. Evan told about his reasons for coming as a refugee, the dangers he faced, and his determination to protect his family by hiding himself, distancing himself from them, and ultimately deciding he must leave his and their country. He spoke of his ability to triumph over the "isolation and despair."

JH: At any time did you find yourself questioning your values about the importance of your family that led you to come here, or even the values that were important to you politically? Did this cause you to question that, or did you hang on to those?

E: No question. My family is more important than whatever I was trying to do politically. Because for me, family is number one.

JH: Yeah. So, way more than what you were interested in politically, was the fact that you came here in order to preserve your family. . . . So what kept you here was your love for your family? That, however difficult it was, you knew you were making the right decision?

E: Right.

JH: Is that something that you would tell yourself?

E: Yes, well I always said, "I have to do this." And I remember my Mom always said, I'm a warrior. That's what she said; that I'm a warrior. So . . . now that I think about it, I guess I said to myself, "I am a warrior . . . I'm going to do it."

JH: So this was your way of being a warrior for your family?

E: Yes! I was and I still am.

The description of himself as a "warrior" was in the background, but not fully known to Evan until this conversation. Now it is more available to him as an image or metaphor to rely on.

As we have observed clinically, we expected that these single sessions, which were designed to invoke novelty, naming, enthusiasm, social engagement, and optimal arousal would result in observable differences in cortisol, alpha-amylase and EEG readings. At the time of the writing of this chapter, we have analyzed results from a cohort of 20 participants, 10 in the neutral situation and 10 in the narrative situation. We are completing the collection and analysis of an additional five in each group.

Our results show statistically different patterns on both biomarkers, with the neutral group showing no noticeable response to the conversations, and the single session narrative conversations showing increases in these markers of social engagement across the conversations. The EEG results suggested, but did not conclusively demonstrate, that alpha waves, a marker of calm engagement, showed no change across time for the neutral group, but increased over the course of the session for the narrative group. In other words, despite a very small sample, we saw biological effects on markers of social engagement over the narrative conversations. We hope and expect that the next data analysis will show the same for alpha wave measures as well. It appears that it is possible to demonstrate that scaffolding-based brief narrative conversations have neurophysiological effects, consistent with ideas proposed from the perspective of interpersonal neurobiology (Cozolino, 2010; Siegel, 2012).

Implications for Our Clinical Work and Teaching

Karen and Jim are each practicing and teaching within an ever-increasing world of evidence-based practices. With the increasing popularity of the use of collaborative therapies, and specifically brief narrative practices within single session and walk-in therapy, there is a demand for evidence of the effectiveness of these practices. This research therefore is timely as it confirms neurophysiological effects of brief therapeutic encounters with people. This confirmatory evidence has impacted our brief therapy practices. It helps us to remain dedicated to a single session therapy that is highly socially engaging as we generate details and rich novel descriptions of problems and initiatives in people's lives. We each teach therapists who are training in single session contexts about the importance of co-developing unique and personally meaningful names for the problems that impact people's lives. We highlight that single session therapy needs to include powerfully moving language development and connection to what people are proud of and prefer in their lives and how they might move toward these. Both of us, in our teaching and supervision, refer to our research findings that support the measureable neurophysiological effects of these conversations as demonstrating the socially engaging nature of brief narrative practices guiding single session therapy. We remind therapists that generating curiosity, enthusiasm, collaboration, and optimal arousal in single sessions creates a high degree of social engagement, a condition that is essential for impactful therapeutic encounters.

References

Arita H. (2012). Anterior prefrontal cortex and serotonergic system activation during Zen meditation practice induces negative mood improvement and increased alpha in EEG. *Rinsho Shinkeigaku*, 52(11), 1279–1280.

Badenoch, B. (2011). *The brain-savvy therapist's workbook*. New York, NY: W. W. Norton & Company Inc.

Beaudoin, M. N. (2010). *The SKILL-ionaire in every child: Boosting children's socio-emotional skills using the latest in brain research*. San Francisco: Goshawk Publications.

Beaudoin, M.-N., & Zimmerman, J. (2011). Narrative therapy and interpersonal neurobiology: Revisiting classic practices, developing new emphases. *Journal of Systemic Therapies, 48*(1), 1–13.

Cozolino, L. (2010). *The neuroscience of psychotherapy: Healing the social brain* (2nd ed.). New York, NY: W. W. Norton & Company Inc.

Duvall, J., & Young, K. (2009). Keeping the faith: A conversation with Michael White. *Journal of Systemic Therapies, 28*(1), 1–18.

Duvall, J., & Young, K. (2015). Brief Services: Foundational Principles and Therapeutic Approaches. Online Course, www.complexneeds.ca

Duvall, J., Young, K., & Kayes-Burden, A. (2012). No more, no less: Brief mental health services for children and youth. Retrieved from www.excellence forchildandyouth.com

Hanson, R., & Mendius, R. (2009). *Buddha's brain.* Oakland, CA: New Harbinger Publishers.

Hibel, L. C., Trumbell, J. M., & Mercado, E. (2014). Work/non-workday differences in mother, child, and mother-child morning cortisol in a sample of working mothers and their children. *Early Human Development, 90*, 1–7.

Howells, F.M., Ives-Deliperi, V.L., Horn, N.R., & Stein, D.J. (2012). Mindfulness based cognitive therapy improves frontal control in bipolar disorder: A pilot EEG study. *BM Psychiatry, 29*, 12–15.

Hubble, M. A., Duncan, B. L., & Miller, S. D. (1999). *The heart & soul of change: What works in therapy.* Washington, DC: American Psychological Association.

Lambert, M. J., Shapiro, D. A., & Bergin, A. E. (1994). The effectiveness of psychotherapy. In S. L. Garfield & A. E. Bergin (Eds.), *Handbook of psychotherapy and behavior change* (pp. 157–211). New York, NY: John Wiley & Sons Inc. (Original work published in 1986).

Lutz, A., McFarlin, D.R., Perlman D.M., Salomons, T.V, & Davidson, R. J. (2013). Altered anterior insula activation during anticipation and experience of painful stimuli in expert meditators. *Neuroimage, 1*(64), 538–546.

Maclennan, R. (2015). Co-creating pivotal moments: Narrative practice and neuroscience. *Journal of Systemic Therapies, 34*(1), 43–60.

Miskovic, V., Moscovitch, D. A., Santesso, D. L., McCabe, R. E., Antony, M. M., & Schmidt L. A. (2011). Changes in EEG cross-frequency coupling during cognitive behavioral therapy for social anxiety disorder. *Psychological Science, 22*(4), 507–516.

Moscovitch, D. A., Santesso, D. L., Miskovic, V., McCabe, R. E., Antony, M. M., & Schmidt, L. A. (2011). Frontal EEG asymmetry and symptom response to cognitive behavioral therapy in patients with social anxiety disorder. *Biological Psychology, 87*(3) 379–385.

Orlinsky, D. E., Grawe, K., & Parks, B. K. (1994). Process and outcome in psychotherapy. In A. E. Bergin & S. L. Garfield (Eds.), *Handbook of psychotherapy and behavior change* (pp. 270–376). New York, NY: John Wiley & Sons Inc.

Ramey, H. L., Young, K., & Tarulli, D. (2010). Scaffolding and concept formation in narrative therapy: A qualitative research report. *Journal of Systemic Therapies, 29*(4), 74–91.

Shirtcliff, E., Peres, J., Dismukes, A., Lee, Y., & Phan, J. (2014). Riding the physiological roller coaster: Adaptive significance of cortisol stress reactivity to social contexts. *Journal of Personality Disorders, 28*(1), 40–51.

Siegel, D. J. (2011). *Mindsight: The new science of personal transformation.* New York, NY: Bantam Books.

Siegel, D. J. (2012). *Pocket guide to interpersonal neurobiology: An integrative handbook of the mind.* New York, NY: W. W. Norton & Company Inc.

Siegel, D., & Bryson, T. P. (2012). *The Whole-Brain Child: 12 Revolutionary strategies to nurture you child's developing mind.* California: Mind Your Brain, Inc.

Siegel, D. J., & Payne, B. T. (2012). *The whole brain child.* New York, NY: Bantam Books Trade Paperbacks.

Sobolewski, A., Holt, E., Kublik, E., & Wróbel, A. (2011). Impact of meditation on emotional processing—a visual ERP study. *Neuroscience Research, 71*(1), 44–48.

Vygotsky, L. S. (1978). *Mind in society: The development of higher psychological processes* (Ed. M. Cole, V. John-Steiner, S. Scribner, & E. Souberman). Cambridge, MA: Harvard University Press.

Vygotsky, L. S. (1987). Thinking and speech. In R. W. Rievery & A. S. Carton (Eds.) & N. Minnick (Trans.), *The collected works of L. S. Vygotsky, Volume 1: Problems of general psychology* (pp. 39–285). New York, NY: Plenum Press.

White, M. (1989). Negative explanation, restraint, & double description: A template for family therapy. In M. White (Ed.), *Selected papers* (pp. 85–99). Adelaide, South Australia: Dulwich Centre Publications.

White, M. (2006). Externalizing conversations revisited. In A. Morgan & M. White (Eds.), *Narrative therapy with children and their families* (pp. 2–56). Adelaide, South Australia: Dulwich Centre Publications.

White, M. (2007). *Maps of narrative practice.* New York, NY: W. W. Norton & Company Inc.

Young, K. (2008). Narrative practice at a walk-in therapy clinic: Developing children's worry wisdom. *Journal of Systemic Therapies, 27*(4), 54–74.

Young, K. (2011a). When all the time you have is now: Re-visiting practices and narrative therapy in a walk-in clinic. In J. Duvall & L. Béres (Eds.), *Innovations in narrative therapy: Connecting practice, training, and research* (pp. 147–166). New York, NY: W. W. Norton & Company Inc.

Young, K. (2011b). Narrative practices at a walk-in therapy clinic. In A. Slive & M. Bobele (Eds.), *When one hour is all you have: Effective therapy for walk-in clients* (pp. 149–166). Phoenix, AZ: Zeig, Tucker & Theisen.

Zimmerman, J., & Beaudoin, M.-N. (2015). Neurobiology for your narrative: How brain science can influence narrative work. *Journal of Systemic Therapies, 34*(2), 59–74.

9 Neuroscience Discourse and the Collaborative Therapies?

Tom Strong

In this chapter I approach interpersonal neurobiology and its applications to a collaborative psychotherapy as an emergent yet influential discourse of practice. Neuroscience discourse, for me, refers to science-informed understandings and practices that privilege the mind (often understood as the brain) as the primary seat of human action and understanding, extended to include the interpersonal neurobiology of Daniel Siegel (2012). The promises of neuroscience got President Obama's financial backing and advocacy (2013), while attracting a considerable critical response (e.g., Busso & Pollack, 2015; Rose & Abi-Rached, 2013). Though still at a kind of frontier, "brain-based" learning (e.g., Busso & Pollack, 2015) and therapy (e.g., Beaudoin & Zimmerman, 2011; Cozolino & Santos, 2014; Schore, 2012) have become common and publicly accepted applications of neuroscience discourse.

My Relationship with Neuroscience

This chapter began from a conversation with co-editor, Marie-Nathalie over Peter Hacker's concerns about the pros and cons of neuroscience (in Bennett, Dennett, Hacker, & Searle, 2007). Hacker warned of a "mereological fallacy," the increasingly popular notion that brain parts have agency (i.e., make things happen on their own), as indicated by oddly grammatical yet not uncommon statements such as the following: Susie's frontal lobes (amygdala, etc.) *manage* the social situation she is in. I am a social constructionist, theory nerd (e.g., Lock & Strong, 2010) interested in why conversations should make a difference in clients' lives. Non-constructionists (many in neuroscience I discovered) dismiss this view as "folk psychology" (Churchland & Haldane, 1988) and focus instead on scientifically "correct" understandings, about which I am wary. Two strands of discourse analysis (see Woofitt, 2005) informed my read of the neuroscience literature: the critical discourse tradition drawing from Foucault (1973) and the micro-interactional tradition of conversation analysts. "Features" refer to how aspects of neuroscience discourse are described while "practices" refer to how these features might be used in collaborative therapy. These features/practices vary in the literature, so I will highlight how they vary using binaries: 1) singular/multiple explanatory discourses, 2) hard-wiring/sedimenting, 3) brain-based/dialogical explanations of agency and change, 4) and brainfulness/mindfulness.

Singular/Multiple Explanatory Discourses?

Most collaborative therapists work *within* clients' languages (e.g., Anderson, 1997), without correcting or discounting clients' languages of understanding with expert discourse. Thus, a challenge in using neuroscience discourse may be to find ways to use and supplement neuroscience understandings without invoking hierarchical linguistic expertise. To illustrate, injury can be understood as more than a biomedical phenomenon; it acquires different and added meanings in our relationships, work, aspirations, and so on.

Sometimes neuroscience discourse presents explanations as singular and foundational for understanding and acting: "Discovering the biological mechanisms underlying social interactions is one of the major problems for the interdisciplinary field of neuroscience to address in the twenty-first century" (Norman, Hawkley, Cole, Berntson, & Cacioppo, 2012, p. 89). What rhetorical or conversational purpose might such a straightforward explanation aim to accomplish, a discourse analyst might ask? One might start by examining the language or linguistic resources used, such as metaphor (Gotman, 2012; Lakoff & Johnson, 1980). Two common neuroscience discourse metaphors jump out in this sentence: "biological mechanisms" and "underlying." A common machine metaphor is used in cognitive psychology and the media: our brains *are* information-processing computers with yet-to-be-discovered, or possibly faulty, software or hardware (cf. Marcus, June 27, 2015). A more rhetorically powerful metaphor in this quote reassures us that underlying mechanisms may be discoverable and inevitably modifiable. While I may seem to single out Norman and colleagues (above), neuroscience discourse often singularly and mechanically conveys that understanding and acting are brain functions alone.

Another singular species of brain-based discourse promises "O" objectivity for new subdisciplines, such as neuroethics, neuro education, and neuro economics, presumably enabling human affairs to be conducted objectively and rationally (cf. Pickersgill, 2013). The underlying thrust in these new disciplines, for critics, is to super-impose a particular rationality (male, exploitative, etc.) by optimizing particular brain parts, processes, and pursuit of outcomes in the name of that rationality. There can be a "here's what is really going on and what should be done" logic often at work in the subdisciplines taking up this subdiscourse (Ortega & Vidal, 2011).

Neuroscience is increasingly informing expert medical discourse; such as when accounting for mental disorders, such as ADHD (Conrad, 2007). Neuroscience understandings, like most forms of expert medical discourse, also become accessible through popular and self-help media, offering prospective clients a legitimizing language people can "grow into" (Hacking, 2006; Racine & Costa-van Aesch, 2011; Rose & Abi-Rached, 2013)—a challenge for therapists conversing in clients' languages. Translated to therapy, a focus on getting the right explanation (i.e., a "differential diagnosis") can come with a cost, however. Understandably, a binary logic (right/wrong, Thomas & Bracken, 2011) can emerge for therapist or client where a neuroscience explanation preclude others. Such expert discourse may tilt conversation to therapist expertise over therapy's correct terms or understandings, potentially usurping collaborative aspects of a "client is expert" participation (Anderson & Goolishian, 1992).

The eighteenth-century philologist Vico (2005/1744) wrote of "linguistic poverty"—a lack of helpful alternative or supplementary understandings and discourses (i.e., discursive resources). Neuroscience discourse and its related understandings afford some reassuring understandings without requiring foreclosure on alternative discourses or meanings. Collaborative therapists tend to flexibly host conversations, using varied discursive resources to make sense of and address client concerns (Strong, 2016). At a minimum, neuroscience discourse need not narrow track therapeutic dialogue—it can be supplemented by other discourses or discursive resources to add understandings that enable alternative courses of action (Gergen, 2015).

My interest in neuroscience discourse and its use in therapy arises from examining how therapist and client negotiate a recognizably shared language and conversational process for their work together (e.g., Strong & Pyle, 2012). This research adapted the micro-interactional focus of conversation analysts (Pain, 2009) and discursive psychologists (Edwards & Potter, 1992) to understand how turns and sequences of conversation are negotiated between client and therapist. My concern had been that, while collaborative therapists talked about the importance of conversation, few studied it using conversational methods of research (exception, Gale & Newfeld, 1992). The focus of these research methods is on how people take their turns at dialogue, responding to therapy's conversational junctures, in ways that illustrate how neuroscience discourse, for example, might be taken up, or not.

Turning to a fictional client, George sought therapy, at his partner's suggestion. He has not been himself, he says, and wants to get to the bottom of what may be wrong so that he can get back on the right track. He recently watched a TV show about the brain's executive functions and neuroplasticity (e.g., Doidge, 2015) and "knows that depression runs in [his] family." George, however, also has experienced some chronic pain issues, and major upheavals within his work that have translated into an uncertain financial future. Above all, he wants to find out what is wrong so he can get on with making things right. Conversant in neuroscience as well as other therapeutic discourses, George's therapist reviews the combination of things that may have prompted George to come in for

therapy, including his interest in neuroplasticity. The conversational juncture they must work out next in talking and listening begins here:

George: Sure, I can appreciate other things adding to my stress and
             potential for depression, but what is wrong with my execu-
             tive functioning, and does it affect how I am feeling?
Therapist: . . .

Wary of any discourse's capacity to "capture" (Massumi, 2011) or dominate, collaborative therapists can face a balancing act of welcoming what
clients present, while possibly negotiating supplements to (or reflection
on) the constraints of any singular discourse. George seems to expect
his therapist to restrict her dialogue to a neuroscience discourse focused
on executive functioning. What might such an exclusive focus mean for
their dialogue? The usual response of collaborative therapists is a kind of
yes/and to such client expectations; welcome what clients present and, if
what they hear is not what they want to endorse or extend, negotiate the
conversational process and content elsewhere in ways clients can accept.
Such a negotiation will not occur over one turn of talking; junctures
like the above call for discursive awareness and resourcefulness (Strong,
2016). Discursive awareness relates to recognizing how language is used
and in recognizing potential dialogue openings at such junctures, while
discursive resourcefulness refers to how our responses in such openings
can extend or negotiate alternatives to any discourse. If knowledgeable
and conversant in neuroscience discourse, the obvious response is to offer
George the neuroscience explanation he seeks. However, discourses are
more than neutral groupings of words: they extend particular logics and
values to understand and act from. Responding to George's upsets as
brain-based, as part of his executive functioning, would acknowledge
his present discourse; however, suppose the therapist wants to invite and
negotiate a more discursively resourceful dialogue? For now, consider the
questions below:

a) What resources does neuroscience discourse offer you and your cli-
    ents that didn't exist before neuroscience?
b) Singular discourses (certainties?) are most common when emotional
    and other stakes are high; where are they most common in your and
    your clients' understandings and ways of communicating?
c) How do you introduce further discourses where a singular client dis-
    course of understanding and communicating has held sway?

Brain-Based/Dialogical Agency: Do Brains Have Minds of Their Own?

Neuroscience discourse is commonly used to explain varied phenomena
as "brain-based." While usually innocuous, such as humans are "wired to

connect with others" (e.g., De Koven Fishbane, 2013, Kindle Location, 131), this discourse is often replete with claims of what brains "allow" or "control"—claims Satel and Lillienfeld (2013) see as "mindless brain science." Still, it is not uncommon to hear or read of brain parts single-mindedly doing, causing, allowing, etc., which is not unlike saying my knee took me out for a walk.

Brain-based agency is a neuroscience subdiscourse that locates agency (our ability to intend or make things happen) in brain parts and bio-chemical processes in the brain, and not in a mindedness that extends beyond the brain (e.g., Noë, 2009; Putnam, 1981, evocatively wrote decades earlier of a "brain in a vat"). Most neuroscientists do not claim that brains or brain parts act as isolated, intentional agents (cf. Coulter, 1979); they write in associationist or correlationist terms (when engaged in mental activity, brain part or process X is activated). Problems arise when intentions or independent actions are ascribed to these correlated parts or processes. While FMRI brain scans show activated parts and processes, for Dumit (2004), brain imagery has identity-shaping implications, conveying what our brains seemingly do irrespective of our experiences and actions. Such images offer corroborating evidence helpfully showing what parts and processes of the brain get used in activities, particularly useful if there are underdeveloped or injured aspects of the brain. By analogy, like muscles I had to retrain after getting a titanium knee, one can engage in activities that "boost" (Beaudoin, 2014) one's brain power to better do particular mental activities. In the interpersonal neurobiology discourse of authors such as Louis Cozolino (2010), one reads of social brains, or that empathy is brain-based. There is no chicken or egg here. While our brains do not *cause* our love or social lives, our capacity for sociality or love is strengthened by engaging in those activities which, *concurrently*, engage brain parts or processes that are not brain-encapsulated.

Many intelligent interactive processes start as challenging and awkward before being performed elegantly in taken-for-granted or tacit ways (Dreyfus & Dreyfus, 1987; Polanyi, 1966). Further, many "intelligent" interactions and processes occur implicitly within our bodies (brain included) without our awareness: circulating blood, digesting food, growing hair, and so on. For Hubert Dreyfus (1991), much of our "being-in-the-world" happens tacitly (in taken-for-granted ways) and it is only in experiencing failures with or disruptions to such tacit acts that we are jarred back to having to deal with them in more explicit and intentional ways. Helping clients recognize that particular interactions have a greater chance of recurring because they also concurrently activate brain processes is different from suggesting that their brains are responsible for empathy or sharing. Returning to George, given this discussion of brain-based agency, I ask readers to imagine the conversation further along, after discussing links between his upsets and executive functioning. In rejoining their dialogue, George presents an initial mereological claim:

George: So, problems with my executive functioning cause the argu-
           ments I have at home?
Therapist: In part yes . . .

While clearly a simplistic exaggeration of brain-based agency subdis-course, this juncture invites consideration of where and how such a sub-discourse may come up short for client and therapist.

Building on narrative ideas from James Griffiths's and Melissa Griffiths's (1994) *The Body Speaks,* I long ago became interested in intersections of the biological and the circumstantial (Strong, 1997), especially their views on how clients could "partner" with medications to optimize preferred outcomes. While brain-based accounts of agency can help to move understanding out of a morally questioned realm (e.g., George gets upset because he is bad), they may offer incomplete explanations where further actionable understandings may be possible. Assuming George is ok with the therapist's "In part yes . . ." response above, and perhaps a few conversational turns down the line, a thera-pist could introduce supplements such as those following: When does executive functioning have the greatest influence over the upsets and when do the upsets have the greatest influence on your executive func-tioning? When do you and executive functioning best work together in keeping upsets in their place? Here are some further reflective questions to ponder: a) In your own theories of problems and solutions, how central is the brain or mental processes to those theories? b) How have you integrated neuroscience understandings into how you account for stability and change in clients' lives? c) What role do our interactions with others and aspects of physical reality play in stability and change, beyond our brains?

Hard-Wiring/Sedimenting/Stabilizing: Enduring Changes through Repetition?

Related to repeated neuronal firing (Hebb's, 1949 mantra: neurons that fire together wire together) is a phenomenon Ricoeur (1977) described as "sedimenting" meanings and discourse. Geologists similarly describe how successive deposits of soil become stable as rock. A focus on stabi-lizing meaning and action, from what had been random and uninten-tional to becoming intentionally re-producible, featured in Vygotsky's (1978) sociocultural approach to learning. While we can learn to make spontaneous and otherwise random actions occur deliberately, deliberate action over time is needed to stabilize new and preferred interactions. Regardless of how meanings and actions become reproducibly familiar, stabilizing or sedimenting them can relate not only to how neurons fire together, but to how we make new interactions habitual.

Brain-boosting activities analogous to physical fitness training or rehabilitation have been developed to enhance or rehabilitate mental performances—to stabilize desired mental processes where they are new, or have lapsed or been disrupted (Beaudoin, 2014). Brain-based explanations add to our understandings of how we become adept at anticipating and responding to recurring developments. This anticipatory dimension of human interaction (Kinsbourne & Jordan, 2009) enables us to sense what might happen next in interactions with others, or with aspects of the physical world. Samuel Todes (2001) referred to this anticipatory dimension as *poise*, or our ability to be responsive to a range of developments normally occurring in and from our interactions. Such poise is seen in tennis professionals, good dancers, and veteran pilots, and reflects both inner (i.e., brain processes) and outer (i.e., patterned interactions) correlates that can be understood as competence. Evidence from neuroscience highlights how inner brain processes are stabilized as clients acquire poise for reliably responding to outer learning and interpersonal challenges, thickening and sedimenting a client's story of change.

In continuing with George, it would not be uncommon to hear something like:

George: I hear a lot of good ideas but none of them seem to stick with me after leaving therapy.

Many neuroscience-informed therapists see such a conversational opening, for George, as helpful for anticipating upsets for which he could sediment new executive functioning practices, or strengthen new neuronal connections. Anticipatable problems, in narrative therapy terms, have "rules" or "requirements" for their perpetuation (Doan & Clifton, 1990). Once such "rules" are known, new practices can be introduced and then sedimented (i.e., practiced until habitual) through repetition in ways highlighted by Beaudoin (2014) with kids and De Koven Fishbane (2013) with adults in couples. Some questions to stimulate further therapist reflection on these points might be: a) In your theory of therapeutic change, to what extent have you factored in repetition of change behaviors as part of the change process? b) What do you presently do in your work with clients to stabilize or sediment change? c) How do you explain "neuroplasticity" to clients given that making and stabilizing client-preferred changes can seem so challenging?

Brainfulness and Mindfulness: Locating Intelligence and Wellbeing

Notions of what is meant by "mental" or "mindful" have been shifting in recent decades. Gregory Bateson (1972) asked, for example, if a blind person's cane, for being so intricately interwoven with that person's perceptual abilities and related movements, was part of that blind person's mindfulness. A growing public acceptance relates interpersonal neurobiology to an expanded sense of "mindfulness," particularly among neuroscience-informed educators and therapists, as well as practitioners of mindfulness meditation (e.g., Kabat-Zinn, 2005; Siegel, 2012). Therapists have long used relaxation to address emotions that disrupt desired performances or ways of being, exemplified by a recent and constructive engagement between Buddhist practices of meditation and cognitive therapy (e.g., Segal, Williams, & Teasdale, 2012). Brain imagery supports how evidence-based practices of mindfulness help in addressing disruptive and excessive emotions. Being mindful increasingly means being perceptually and intellectually engaged in ways associated with clarity and groundedness. Mindfulness practices have been helpful (see the American Mindfulness Research Association website: https://goamra.org/) in reducing emotional upset, feeling more at home in our bodies and circumstances (i.e., grounded), and being able to act with greater awareness and purpose (i.e., clarity).

Mindfulness is arguably a different subdiscourse than brain-based subdiscourse. Critical psychologists and sociologists suggest that brain-focused, attention inward deflects attention away from potentially transformable, external influences on wellbeing (Rose & Abi-Rached, 2013) while assisting pharmaceutical interests aiming to optimize wellbeing through enhanced chemical management (Gergen, 2015). Interpersonal neurobiological descriptions suggest a kind of mindfulness that is situated, process oriented, embodied, contextually responsive, and relational. Instead of seeing specific brain parts or processes as causal, this literature speaks of systemic inter-relationships of parts, processes, external engagements, and other factors. A phenomenologist's sense of subjective experience (what things mean for me, Zahavi, 2008) and agency, however, can seem to drop from view in this interpersonal neurobiological account. A primary therapeutic focus of interpersonal neurobiological mindfulness discourse is on integration, bringing the mental system, inclusive of all its external and internal parts, into coherence or harmony. Consistent with Buddhist outcomes associated with mindfulness practice, Siegel, wrote, "[k]indness is integration made visible" (2012, Kindle Location 2854).

Brainfulness and mindfulness are clearly different subdiscourses, though they can sometimes become problematically conflated (e.g., "Oxytocin *allows us* to put down our weapons and engage, to bond, procreate and raise our young" De Koven Fishbane, 2013 Kindle location, 1384, italics added). More commonly however, collaborative therapists seek to promote mindful integration within coherent client life narratives (Zimmerman & Beaudoin, 2015). This is not always how clients come to understand mindfulness, as George highlights.

George: (referring to his therapist's mention of their possibly using mindfulness practices) You are not going to try to make me into a Buddhist now, are you?

Most therapists have their ways of introducing interventions and a rationale for supporting their use in therapy. There is an evidence base supporting the use of neuroscience-based interventions to enhance mindfulness practice in therapy (Cozolino & Santos, 2014; Schore, 2012). Addressing upsets is one such focus of mindfulness practice, a way to de-stress and better attune body, mind, and circumstances (Kabat-Zinn, 2005). Thus, George's quip in the conversational juncture above can readily be met with a therapist response regarding the science supporting mindfulness practices. Should he accept such a rationale, George could learn, with practice (i.e., sedimenting) how to use his executive functioning to "tune in," to relate to both his internal experience and external circumstances associated with the upsets he has been experiencing (Siegel, 2012). However, therapists as well as clients can have questions regarding the applicability of the growing range of mindfulness practices for addressing concerns beyond clients' internal experiences: a) How do you understand and facilitate mindfulness in therapy? b) What parts of practicing collaborative therapy are enhanced by use of neuroscience discourse, and possibly distracted by this discourse? c) Interpersonal neurobiology brings together relational and mental processes. How do you see these processes as integrated and/or separate?

Discussion

Throughout this chapter, I have focused on particular features and uses (or practices) I see associated with neuroscience discourse. I think any discourse both affords and constrains possibilities for understanding and action. I also wonder about our abilities to avoid the trap that critical discourse analysts and theorists (Fairclough, 1990; Foucault, 1973) identify clearly: that we tend to gravitate to singular discourses that dominate or act as default understandings—again affording some possibilities while constraining others. Biological discourse—neuroscience or interpersonal neurobiology included—is still discourse, a human construction we can use with flexibility and resourcefulness (Dingwall, Nerlich, & Hillyard, 2003). I personally find it helpful that neuroscience evidence supports practices I use as a collaborative therapist, such as those I have been describing here when considering: 1) singular/multiple discourses, 2) brain-based/dialogical agency and change, 3) hard-wiring/sedimenting, and 4) brainfulness/mindfulness. Through conversational junctures, such as those "George" brought us to in his therapy, binaries or dilemmas can emerge in ways that can, conversationally speaking, put therapists on the spot. So my aim here has been to critically focus on aspects of neuroscience discourse that might feel at odds with ways collaborative therapists think about their conversational practice with clients. In my own approach to practice (Strong, 2016), my focus has been on discursive awareness and discursive resourcefulness: recognizing how therapists' and clients' language use affords and constrains therapy's possibilities. Neuroscience discourse clearly adds a useful discourse for practicing collaborative therapy, if turned to with such awareness and resourcefulness.

References

American Mindfulness Research Association. (n.d.). Retrieved from https://goamra.org/

Anderson, H. (1997). *Conversation, language, and possibilities.* New York, NY: Basic Books.

Anderson, H., & Goolishian, H. (1992). The client is the expert: A not knowing approach to therapy. In S. McNamee & K. Gergen (Eds.), *Therapy as social construction* (pp. 25–39). Newbury Park, CA: Sage.

Bateson, G. (1972). *Steps to an ecology of mind.* New York, NY: Ballantyne.

Beaudoin, M.-N. (2014). *Boosting all children's social and emotional brain power: Life transforming activities.* Thousand Oaks, CA: Corwin Press.

Beaudoin, M.-N., & Zimmerman, J. (2011). Narrative therapy and interpersonal neurobiology: Revisiting classic practices, developing new emphases. *Journal of Systemic Therapies, 30*(1), 1–13.

Bennett, M., Dennett, D., Hacker, P., & Searle, J. (2007). *Neuroscience & philosophy: Brain, mind, & language.* New York, NY: Columbia University Press.

Busso, D. S., & Pollack, C. (2015). No brain left behind: Consequences of neuroscience discourse for education. *Learning, Media and Technology, 40,* 168–186.

Churchland, P., & Haldane, J. (1988). Folk psychology and the explanation of human behavior. *Proceedings of the Aristotelian Society, 62,* 209–221.

Conrad, P. (2007). *The medicalization of society: On the transformation of human conditions into treatable disorders.* Baltimore, MD: Johns Hopkins University Press.

Coulter, J. (1979). The brain as agent. *Human Studies, 2,* 335–348.

Cozolino, L. J. (2010). *The neuroscience of psychotherapy: Healing the social brain* (2nd ed.). New York, NY: W. W. Norton & Company Inc.

Cozolino, L. J., & Santos, E. N. (2014). Why we need therapy—and why it works: A neuroscientific perspective. *Smith College Studies in Social Work, 84,* 157–177.

De Koven Fishbane, M. (2013). *Loving with the brain in mind: Neurobiology and couple therapy.* New York, NY: W. W. Norton & Company Inc.

Dingwall, R., Nerlich, B., & Hillyard, S. (2003). Biological determinism and symbolic interaction: Hereditary streams and cultural roads. *Symbolic Interaction, 26,* 631–644.

Doan, R., & Clifton, D. (1990). The rules of problem lifestyles: Making externalizations more real. *Dulwich Centre Newsletter, 4*(1), 18–21.

Doidge, N. (2015). *The brain's way of healing: Remarkable discoveries and recoveries from the frontiers of neuroplasticity.* New York, NY: Viking.

Dreyfus, H. L. (1991). *Being-in-the-world: A commentary on Heidegger's being and time, division 1*. Cambridge, MA: MIT Press.

Dreyfus, H. L., & Dreyfus, S. E. (1987). *Mind over machine: The power of human intuition and expertise in the era of the computer*. New York, NY: Free Press.

Dumit, J. (2004). *Picturing personhood: Brain scans and biomedical identity*. Princeton, NJ: Princeton University Press.

Edwards, D., & Potter, J. (1992). *Discursive psychology*. Thousand Oaks, CA: Sage.

Fairclough, N. (1990). *Language and power*. London, UK: Longman.

Foucault, M. (1973). *The order of things: An archaeology of the human sciences*. New York, NY: Vintage.

Gale, J., & Newfeld, N. (1992). A conversation analysis of solution-focused marital therapy session. *Journal of Marital and Family Therapy, 18*, 153–165.

Gergen, K. J. (2015). The neurobiological turn in therapeutic treatment: Salvation or devastation? In D. Loewenthal (Ed.), *Critical psychotherapy, psychoanalysis and counselling: Implications for practice* (pp. 53–73). London, UK: Palgrave Macmillan.

Gotman, K. (2012). The neural metaphor. In M. M. Littlefield & J. Jenell (Eds.), *Neuroscientific turn: Transdisciplinarity in the age of the brain* (pp. 71–86). Ann Arbor, MI: University of Michigan Press.

Griffiths, J. L., & Griffiths, M. E. (1994). *The body speaks: Therapeutic dialogues for mind-body problems*. New York, NY: Basic Books.

Hacking, I. (2006). Kinds of people: Moving targets. *Proceedings of the British Academy, 151*, 285–315.

Hebb, D. O. (1949). *The organization of behavior*. New York, NY: John Wiley & Sons.

Kabat-Zinn, J. (2005). *Coming to our senses: Healing ourselves and the world through mindfulness*. New York, NY: Hachette Books.

Kinsbourne, M., & Jordan, J. S. (2009). Embodied anticipation: A neurodevelopmental interpretation. *Discourse Processes, 46*(2), 103–126.

Lakoff, G., & Johnson, M. (1980). *Metaphors we live by*. Chicago, IL: University of Chicago Press.

Lock, A., & Strong, T. (2010). *Social constructionism: Sources and stirrings in theory and practice*. New York, NY: Cambridge University Press.

Marcus, G. (2015, June 27). Face it, your brain is a computer. *New York Times*. Retrieved June 28, 2015 from http://www.nytimes.com/2015/06/28/opinion/sunday/face-it-your-brain-is-a-computer.html

Massumi, B. (2011). *Semblance and event: Activist philosophy and the occurrent arts*. Cambridge, MA: MIT Press.

Noë, A. (2009). *Out of our heads: Why you are not your brain, and other lessons from the biology of consciousness*. New York, NY: Hill & Wang.

Norman, G. J., Hawkley, L. C., Cole, S. W., Berntson, G. G., & Cacioppo, J. T. (2012). Social neuroscience: The social brain, oxytocin, and health. *Social Neuroscience, 7*(1), 18–29.

Obama, B. (2013). The White House brain initiative. Retrieved March 15, 2015 from https://www.whitehouse.gov/BRAIN

Ortega, F., & Vidal, F. (Eds.). (2011). *Neurocultures: Glimpses into an expanding universe*. Frankfurt am Main, Germany: Peter Lang.

Pain, J. (2009). *Not just talking: Conversational analysis, Harvey Sacks' gift to therapy*. London, UK: Karnac Books.

Pickersgill, M. (2013). The social life of the brain: Neuroscience in society. *Current Sociology, 13*, 322–340.

Polanyi, M. (1966). *The tacit dimension*. Chicago, IL: University of Chicago Press.

Putnam, H. (1981). *Reason, truth, and history*. New York, NY: Cambridge University Press.

Racine, E., & Costa-van Aesch, Z. (2011). Neuroscience's impact on our self-identity: Perspectives from ethics and public understanding. In F. Ortega & F. Vidal (Eds.), *Neurocultures: Glimpses into an expanding universe* (pp. 83–98). Frankfurt am Main, Germany: Peter Lang.

Ricoeur, P. (1977). *The rule of metaphor: Multidisciplinary studies of the creation of meaning-making in language* (Trans. R. Czerny). Toronto, ON: University of Toronto Press.

Rose, N., & Abi-Rached, J. M. (2013). *Neuro: The new brain sciences and the management of the mind*. Princeton, NJ: Princeton University Press.

Satel, S., & Lillienfeld, S. O. (2013). *Brainwashed: The seductive appeal of mindless neuroscience*. New York, NY: Basic Books.

Schore, A. N. (2012). *The science of the art of psychotherapy*. New York, NY: W. W. Norton & Company Inc.

Segal, Z. V., Williams, J. M. G., & Teasdale, J. D. (2012). *Mindfulness-based cognitive therapy for depression* (2nd ed.). New York, NY: Guilford Press.

Siegel, D. (2012). *Pocket guide to interpersonal neurobiology: An integrative handbook of the mind*. New York, NY: W. W. Norton & Company Inc.

Strong, T. (1997). Conversations about conversations on chronic pain and illness: Some assumptions and questions for a one day workshop. *Gecko: The Journal of Deconstruction and Narrative Practice, 2*(1), 45–63.

Strong, T. (2016). Discursive awareness and resourcefulness: Bringing discursive researchers into closer dialogue with discursive therapists? In M. O'Reilly & J. Lester (Eds.), *The Palgrave handbook of adult mental health: Discourse and conversation studies* (pp. 481–501). London, UK: Palgrave Macmillan.

Strong, T., & Pyle, N. R. (2012). Negotiating exceptions to clients' problem discourse in consultative dialogue. *Psychology and Psychotherapy: Theory, Research and Practice, 85*(1), 100–116.

Thomas, P., & Bracken, P. (2011). Dualisms and the myth of mental illness. In M. Rapley, J. Moncrieff, & J. Dillon (Eds.), *De-medicalizing misery: Psychiatry, psychology and the human condition* (pp. 10–26). New York, NY: Palgrave Macmillan.

Todes, S. (2001). *Body and world*. Cambridge, MA: MIT Press.

Vico, G. (2005). *New science* (3rd ed.). London, UK: Penguin Books. (Original work published in 1744).

Vygotsky, L. (1978). *Mind in society: The development of higher psychological processes* (Ed. M. Cole, V. John-Steiner, S. Scribner, & E. Souberman). Cambridge, MA: Harvard University Press.

Woofitt, R. (2005). *Conversation analysis and discourse analysis*. London, UK: Sage.

Zahavi, D. (2008). *Subjectivity and selfhood: Investigating the first person perspective*. Cambridge, MA: Bradford.

Zimmerman, J., & Beaudoin, M.-N. (2015). Neurobiology for your narrative: How brain science can influence narrative work. *Journal of Systemic Therapies, 34*(2), 59–74.

Index

"This text offers the reader the opportunity to experience a pivotal moment in their journey as a systemic therapist informed by modern brain science. As all behavior is understood within its context; neurobiology is an essential component of this context. For those who embrace general systems theory yet fully understand that our behaviors and thoughts are governed by neurology, this book is an essential resource. While we intuitively know the connection between collaborative therapy and neurobiology, this text offers a road map for therapists working with individuals, couples, and families within a clinical setting."

—**Peter D. Bradley, PhD,** Cross Timbers Family
Therapy, pllc; Northcentral University

"By combining the literary sensibility of narratively-oriented practice along with the rigor of neurological investigation, Beaudoin and Duvall have achieved a remarkable marriage of two lenses on therapy. This edited volume contains a treasure trove of material for practitioners curious about the synaptic activity accompanying conversations that make a difference."

—**David Paré, PhD,** full professor of counselling psychology,
University of Ottawa; director, The Glebe Institute, a Centre
for Constructive and Collaborative Practice; author,
Collaborative Practice in Counseling and Psychotherapy

Made in the USA
Columbia, SC
01 October 2022

68469475R00085